To All Our Helpers
Across the Threshold

White Feather Publishing Company
5595 White Feather Way
Placerville, California, 95667
(530) 622-9302
email: whitefeather@directcon.net

Second Printing
March 2004

Printed in the United States of America

ISBN 0-9740413-0-0

Books can be ordered from:

Nancy Poer
5595 White Feather Way
Placerville, California, 95667
(530) 622-9302
email: whitefeather@directcon.net

or

Rudolf Steiner College
9200 Fair Oaks Blvd.
Fair Oaks, CA 95628
bookstore@steinercollege.edu
(916) 961-8729

Thank you.

Cover art by Maulsby Kimball
Art Layout by Nancy Poer and Letty Baumgardner
Graphic Design and Production Layout by Letty Baumgardner

Living Into Dying

A JOURNAL
OF SPIRITUAL AND
PRACTICAL DEATHCARE
FOR FAMILY AND COMMUNITY

Nancy Jewel Poer

TABLE OF CONTENTS

FOREWORD

It is hoped that individuals can by aided by these stories of real life experiences to find ways to care for and give support to their loved ones at the threshold of death and beyond. This work is meant for everyone of all religious faiths. While prayers, rituals and religious beliefs can vary, we are all human and all spiritual individualities belonging to the same great universe.

Each death, and the circumstances surrounding it, is unique. Obviously, some of the possibilities described here would not be appropriate for many situations. However, most people do not know that they have choices in the ways they can care for loved ones at death and this is to inform people of their rights and ways that they may find they will want to approach the threshold when the time comes. These stories hopefully also give a sense of how deeply rewarding such participation can be and how our relationship with our loved ones can continue beyond death. The wish is to support each family to find the appropriate religious services and other rituals to honor their loved ones. There is an extensive bibliography for those who want to do further research into spiritual aspects of death.

Stories have been selected to illustrate the different issues and circumstances one can encounter when caring for loved ones and friends at death. There are examples of giving support for the aging and dying process, involvement of family and children, dying at home and after death care, including vigils and funerals. Actual experiences that occurred with authorities—coroners, morticians, and nursing homes are also included. While there are many fine people working in all the institutions that deal with death and dying, it will become clear we have a long way to go to find more humane ways of caring at death. This is one of the reasons why caring for our dead in family and community is an idea whose time has come.

Many of the stories include Christian funeral services for our family view is a broad, inclusive and non-denominational Christian orientation. For me, the true essence of Christianity is that which can embrace all paths to God. I believe it to be that universal power of forgiveness, healing, transformation and resurrection in this world and the spiritual world that is given for all humanity. It is my hope that all people who believe in the immortality of the human soul and spirit can be supported by these thoughts of a spiritual view of their loved one's crossing.

Sadly, I recognize that due to some of the tragic repressive acts done in the name of Christianity, the word alone can be enough to cause many readers to lay a book aside. I understand, for I am wary of fundamental doctrine from any quarter which implies behind it "we are the only ones and the only way," or a view with complete lack of moral conscience. Our age calls for a healthy sense of freedom for our beliefs.

Yet now the whole world stands on the threshold. Good will not automatically prevail but must be chosen and put into deeds. It is time to re-think, to review creatively and objectively all the world's sacred spiritual heritage to find those truths which can inspire us; to find those powers with which we may choose to unite for our own transformation to a higher consciousness and greater enlightenment for the sake of the future of the human race. It is time to know and strive for the spiritual nature of humanity.

This journal is offered with deep gratitude to all those on this side and across the threshold who have inspired this writing and to all those who allowed their stories to be used in order to help others. In some stories names have been changed.

Special thanks to Rev. Richard Lewis, Meg Gorman, Lee Sturgeon-Day, Linda Sussman, Rahima Baldwin, Judy Blatchford, Letty Baumgardner, Robert Boucher and Marijo Rogers who urged me to complete this and helped with editing. Finally, I certainly could not do my work without my husband, Gordon, whose faithful support of the home has made it possible for me to go into the community to give aid. Thanks also to the continuing inspiration of our six children and their wonderful families, Lauren, Gary, Cameron, Mary, Vivian and Colin Michael, to Elizabeth Kubler-Ross for her encouragement to "carry on her work" and above all to Rudolf Steiner, whose profound spiritual insights have guided me towards understanding the great mysteries of life and death.

Post Script — This book was completed just as the United States was attacked on September 11, 2001, and many people died. It is hoped these spiritual thoughts may give comfort and hope in realizing that those beyond the threshold still remain active in giving us support in our lives just as we give support to them with our love, remembrance, and spiritual striving.

Nancy Jewel Poer, Michaelmas, 2001

TIME OF PREPARATION

Our Home: The Four Gables

THE BEGINNING

My life changed when Mother died. Of course one expects such an event to bring change. But these were new and unexpected changes, the before and after distinguished as cleanly as a book falling into two parts. As soon as she had made the transition, the threshold work began for me, which included two years of caring for bedridden elders who died at home, aiding in community home deaths, and then ultimately becoming a nationwide consultant on the subject. The education was immediate and hands on. It included some professional guidance to master the legalities and care of the body, the practical aspects of home death and the uplifting spiritual realities such work entails. Through it all, I have no doubt I have been guided by my mother's energetic inspiration. But then she was born on the threshold herself, just at the turn of the twentieth century on All Souls' Day, so I guess I shouldn't be too surprised.

Frankly, it is hard to imagine anyone saying as a child that she wants to be an undertaker when she grows up, and I certainly never planned to be one. I simply wanted to help family and friends to be able to die at home and be honored there. I suppose many morticians gravitate to their work because it is a family business, or has the financial stability of a trade where, after all, one never runs out of customers.

That's not to say there weren't intimations in my childhood. I was given to playing Red Cross nurse and would stage elaborate funerals for dead birds, lizards, mice and kittens, and even a large beetle or two. Accompanied by earnest prayers, holes were dug and lined with flower petals, crosses were reverently made, and stones and flowers were placed over the crypt.

When I was twelve, I was riding my horse home and had to go a few miles on a very busy road. Our family dog, Blackout, a small short-legged mutt with an outrageously happy blur of a tail that curved over her back, accompanied me. It was World War II, and our town was filled with young men who were being crammed with fighting skills to go fight a heinous enemy. Life was on the edge. As the little dog and I traveled along the highway, suddenly, and despite my pleading and demanding shouts, Blackout began trotting in the road beside me and was immediately run over by a red convertible careening down the road at drunken speed. Two raucous young service men and their shrieking dates were in the car that killed her. They never even looked back. Blinded with tears I struggled to hold my horse and somehow dashed into the traffic to retrieve her body. A kindly milkman stopped and aided me.

9

He lifted the dear limp and bloodied form up in front of my saddle, and offered further help if I needed it. But I refused and rode the interminable three miles home alternating between tight-jawed rage at the callous death and sobbing. My tears fell wet on the silky fur of her still body; my heart was broken with the loss of the precious companion. It marked the transition from childhood dreams to life's harsh realities.

I wonder at that destiny now for, when my parents retired, they bought a home on that same road no more than a stone's throw from where Blackout died and where, decades later, my mother would die just as suddenly with a heart attack.

In the meantime, I grew up and married a wonderful man. I was soon brought to death's stark threshold again with many miscarriages and the stillbirth of our first born child, a son, leaving my husband and me humbled, heart sore and tentative. But fate had a merry compensation awaiting and soon the children came tumbling into our lives, eventually fulfilling a youthful dream of having a family of six children: three sons and three daughters. At the time of my mother's death our eldest child, Lauren, tall, brown-eyed and compassionate, was at the university studying International Relations and longing to serve in the world. Our oldest son, Gary, quick, handsome, decisive and a charmer with an irresistible grin, had just left home and was eagerly taking up building under the tutelage of a brilliant and innovative artist-architect. The next son, Cameron, a gentle giant of six-foot-five inches, was nearing high school graduation. His genius lay in mechanics, and, under his magic touch, go carts, mini-bikes, motorcycles, cars and hybrid contraptions sprang to life to be roared, spun and raced around our old rose garden, flinging gravel to the winds. Our fifteen-year-old identical twin girls, Mary and Vivian, were athletes, swift as young does and as quick to startle. They alternately teased, dramatized, raged and collapsed in giggles. They biked and ran in the then-new triathlon sport, studied with profound seriousness, and created passionately in music and art. The youngest son, Colin Michael, graced and talented, came years later but was filled with such spontaneous and eager joy for life that he warmed our hearts, and made it plain it was indeed worthwhile to raise yet another child.

Our huge, three story 100-year-old home, once part of a large family country estate, well worn and sagging at the foundations, was long past its glory years, but, during our tenure, it burst vibrantly again with all the comings and goings of life: teenage gatherings, festivals, first proms, and family

drama. I taught a nursery school class there. Outside glorious old trees surrounded the home; giant oaks, sycamores, towering palms, and a magnificent magnolia created a beautiful setting for the successions of horses,
goats, guinea pigs, cats and dogs who shared the seasons with us. The place
was a constant neighborhood happening; life was rich at the Poers. And no
one expected the beloved grandmother, Lola, to die that winter.

Mother's Crossing

Lola loomed large in many people's lives. She was filled with a rare
enthusiasm to live life to its fullest and share the joy with others. Certainly
she was a powerful, loving, albeit intense, tower of strength and creativity in
the lives of her children and grandchildren. She was a robust, vibrant force
swirling through the children's lives, and they truly loved her, a doer with a
sturdy body and work-worn hands. She had the same passion and joy for life
and work on earth as she did for affairs of the spirit. Her hair was wispy and
white, her brow high and broad, and dimples deeply lined her face. She had
a splendid frown and evangelical righteousness in the face of laggardly ways.
Her blue eyes sparkled at once with childish joy and transmuted pain: pain
from her baby girl's death, pain from life's struggles in relationships and consciousness, pain from a deep furrow of melancholy in her soul. But they
shone because she willed the spirit light to shine out of them with her prayer
of enthusiasm for all creation, now and forever more, Amen. She had an
unbelievably tender appreciation of everything.

Lola had been there for the birth of every grandchild. No task was too
great or small. She willingly gave every support to make a warm and tender
welcome for the babies. She and Dad had vigorously kept a mountain home
for forty years, a kind of on-going summer camp for many friends and the
grandchildren. There were dress ups, crafts and hikes, nature walks, camp-
outs and her guidance in teaching them how to work and to carry rightful
pride in work well done. Then she lifted their eyes to the heavens and taught
them the stars.

She had intimations death was coming. A month before it came, she told
me she felt she would not have long to live. When she said that, I mentally
ticked off a list. She had no chronic illness we knew of, no cancer or heart
disease. An accident? No, it wasn't her style. I dismissed it. But her great
strength was fading, and, for the first time ever, at seventy-nine, she talked
about "maybe" getting old. Later, we learned she had told a friend she felt she
could "be more help from the other side."

She died at the end of February of a sudden heart attack following a full day of activity. She had weeded the garden, filled three large trashcans with the debris, cultivated the roses, stocked the house with groceries, and visited an artist friend, and asked to see all his beautiful paintings. She was at home, at sunset, when she willed herself across the threshold with her last deed and uttered the words, "We must go through this!"

Many miles away, I received the phone call from one of her neighbors that my mother had just died. Stunned, I put down the phone and sat on the red carpeted stairs in the entry hall. I gathered five of our children around me and told them Grandma Lola had gone into heaven. We wept and wondered that it had really happened. We held each other in a big family hug.

Six-year-old Colin, the youngest son and grandchild, solemnly received the news. But soon he was dancing in and out of the family hug with shining brown eyes and announcing in an exuberant and emphatic tone, "Grandma died, but she's ALIVE!"

It was more than a mere childish wish. It was like an order, the kind of no-nonsense positive statement my mother would make: "This is the truth of the matter, so don't forget it!" When Lauren came home from work, and we told her the news. Her face blanched in stunned disbelief and she left the room in shock. I longed to follow her, but felt I should give her space. I was astonished when she returned in minutes and declared, "How can I be sad? Grandma is just saying, 'Whoopee!'" And so it went. Amidst our tears and shock, these emphatic statements came in these heart warming responses of all of her grandchildren as well as our friends. The beloved grandmother of ten grandchildren, ranging in age from six to twenty-two, had just died, and the initial response of all of them was basically, "Go for it, Grandma!"

At the time this seemed natural, in keeping with Lola's character, but, in retrospect, I realized how extraordinary it was. Basically the response was that Grandma was okay, she knew what she was doing and where she was going, and there was no question that she loved us all. Seventeen-year-old son, Cameron, put it thus, "You know she is happy there, and she gave a lot of happiness to everyone here. She was a wonderful woman so you just can't be sad about it."

This was certainly not because she hadn't been loved or was not missed or grieved for over time. A young child friend, and she had many, said, "I thought Grandma Lola would always be there—like a rock or a favorite tree."

She left people feeling positive because she had so vigorously lived her spiritual beliefs. Through more than forty years of study on a philosophical path of spiritual science, an all embracing wisdom and knowledge that unites the spiritual in humanity with the spiritual in the universe, she had steadfastly demonstrated her faith in the reality of spiritual existence. She had loved her path, lived it, and passed her unwavering faith and enthusiasm on to family and friends. When she went into the next world, it was a heralded event.

There were immediate needs at her death, of course. My father, nearly ninety, ten years her senior, needed support. Never had he imagined he would outlive her, and he was stunned and disoriented at the sudden departure. I flew down to their home while the children drove the five hundred miles to get there. It was all tremulous and challenging for me. It was as though I'd been chosen for some mighty role in a play and I was not at all ready to take on a leading performance. But the play was going on. Bereft and awed, I felt parts of my being scattered and shattered. I had to scoop them up again to go on, for there was a great hole in my existence where the "Mama force" had exited. Yet, like the children, I knew she was okay. Somehow with her inspiration and the blessing of angels, strength came for the tasks of comforting Dad, arranging the funeral and preparing her life story to give as a eulogy.

The kids were amazing. Gary, with his woodworking artistry immediately began designing and building his grandmother's casket in a neighbor's garage. There was no question that he would do it. It was a work of art and a labor of love. When the rest of the family arrived, each one would go over and help to sand and polish the casket for her. We lined it with pretty cloth and sweet smelling leaves of eucalyptus and juniper. The twins, Mary and Vivian, took colored pencils and paper and artistically made the guest book. Cameron, in a quiet natural way, offered to assist the minister in the service. The family ethic of "see what needs to be done and then do it" flowed through each one as an innate response. The girls could also grasp the creative moments while going through her closets, and made numerous appearances in all sorts of dress-up costumes created from Grandma's old hats, gloves, stylish antique beaded purses, and various gowns. Having provided a wondrous array of dress-ups for the grandchildren all their lives, surely Lola would have loved the natural continuity of their joie de vivre with her wardrobe at her crossing.

Comic relief is invariably a part of such affairs. One of the funniest moments, one that still brings my sister and me to shared laughter, occurred when we were shopping together at a fabric store for just the right royal purple cloth to drape underneath the casket. The perky young store clerk kept asking what we were making. Somehow, we felt it too bizarre to try to explain to her, especially as we giggled and furtively pulled the cloth along the yardage counter, "guesstimating" about how long a casket might be. How could we explain our mirth and high spirits on such an occasion? We finally told the inquisitive clerk it was for a "special art project."

The funeral day came. The purple cloth was in place, and a swirl of color in a beautiful painting glowed behind the rich warm wood of the casket, so proudly made by her grandchildren, who were all confident of her pride in their contributions. Bits of rock, pine cones, and sprays of pine branches were around the casket, and on top was the touching little bouquet of Cecil Brunner roses from my father, just as he had given her on their wedding day over half a century before. I gave her eulogy to a full chapel, and we celebrated her crossing with a solemn Christian Community* sacrament. Guitar and folk songs were led by friends, and later we adjourned to home and food and great stories. A friend said, "I must say I enjoyed your mother's funeral." Later, searching in her effects, we found a list of her instructions asking for the funeral service exactly as we had done it and ending with the words . . . "may the family send me joyfully on my spiritual journey and remember that spiritually I can still communicate with them and be ever helpful to them and they to me."

She has been . . . and is. She left a powerful wave of spiritual faith and joy that I hope to share with you. For her path of spiritual striving became mine as well, giving me spirit vision to take action, concepts out of which I would counsel and console others, and awareness of the spirit presence in all of the experience of life.** I would never underestimate the poignant path and process of grief that is part of the threshold experience, for I have known it well with her passing. My hope is that these stories will help others to know the transcendent power of the spirit moving through sadness and transition, so we can, as Lola would say, know that love can mean "to live life heartily."

With the passing of my dynamic mother, my threshold career began, though I didn't know it at the time. My first work was not long in coming.

*a church offering sacraments for life transitions based on indications of Rudolf Steiner. Membership in the church is not required to receive sacraments.

**Anthroposophy—wisdom of the spirit in human life.

BRINGING A LOVED ONE HOME TO DIE

Grandma Mary Edna Goodman

Grandma twinkled. Everyone agreed on that. Her eyes were small and merry brown, but somehow the smallness concentrated the twinkle so they shown out of her softly wrinkled face with penetrating brilliance. Her cheeks were rosy, her smile hearty and infectious, her giggle utterly spontaneous. Actually she was a giggling champion of sorts. At times, to her great embarrassment, she was swept uncontrollably along in laughter when something tickled her funny bone in completely inappropriate situations. On the other side of her nature she could be owlishly quiet and stoic, not unlike a side of my husband, Gordon, her oldest grandson.

In mid life, Mary Edna was extremely heavy for her short, tiny frame. She had developed cascades of truly wondrous double and triple chins. The grandchildren and great grandchildren called them her "wattles." Grandma patiently tolerated their probing little fingers as they cuddled her folds, like a warm wiggly batch of silly putty, with affectionate fascination. Arthritis in her knees had long given her the rolling gait of a sea captain and the children loved that too. It was all part of the archetypal Grandma she was: buttery plump, all loving and always an advocate for the children's point of view. One growing grandchild accused her of getting fat when she was no longer able to fit on Grandma's ample lap and nestle in the comforting haven of her arms. Neighbor children asked if she could be their grandmother too.

Mary Edna had outlived her husband, both her children and one sister. Only a younger sister remained. It was hard to believe that at birth, she had been a tiny premature two-and-a-half pound baby, warmed in a cotton filled shoe box on the back of a wood stove. Yet after a sickly childhood, she was rarely ill and, as an adult, had nursed many others through the devastating influenza of World War I. She spent years on the Indian reservations in the West where she and her husband, George, ran trading posts. She was often alone for long periods of time. But the isolation, the vast stretches of open desert ringed with red mountains and big skies, suited her. Respected by the Navajo native Americans, she was often asked to their sand painting healing ceremonies, an honor few whites enjoyed. At the end of her long life, she concentrated her nurturing energy on a favorite paraplegic grandson and kept house for him.

This was her occupation when, at ninety-two, she slipped and broke her hip. Surgery was done, but poorly, and she became a fully bed-ridden invalid. Unable to bear the idea of her being in an impersonal nursing home, we took stock, rearranged our lives and brought her home. It was a test for our convictions, but we had made a commitment to share death with our children as an inevitable and natural part of life. We also wanted them to know how important it is to care for the elders at the end.

We ordered the hospital bed, the wheelchair, the potty chair, the gowns, the bed pads, diapers and washrags. As I arranged and counted them, I mentioned to my husband that it was very like fixing a layette for a baby. "No, it isn't!" he answered vehemently, not even wanting to look at such an analogy as it had been only three years since we ended a decade and a half of diapers for our own six children. But the day he found himself driving extra slowly over the bumps when we brought Grandma home from the hospital, with our sixteen-year-old twin daughters cuddled protectively on either side of her, he looked at me sideways and muttered, "You're right, you're right!"

She came to the same sunny room where I had taught nursery and kindergarten for many years. The sheer magenta curtains warmed the walls with a rosy glow. It was close by the kitchen where she could easily be attended by the family and be in the flow of life. It seemed very right she should come into this space dedicated to warm beginnings for young children when she had so faithfully been there for the little ones all her life.

The fall and subsequent surgery had weakened and disoriented her, and her consciousness often moved across the borders of ordinary reality. On good days she was up at the family table or out on the porch in her wheelchair. The children tenderly brushed her hair or would bring her savory tidbits between meals. They would often dangle a fake tarantula before her because she would always squeal with such wonderful mock fright. Then they would all laugh together and hug. Some days they would wheel her out with strong youthful arms into the sunshine and bring flowers to fill her lap.

At times she had lightheaded spells where she felt she was dying. Once she called us all to her bedside, and we rushed to gather around. Some of the children brought hastily gathered flowers. We took hands around her bed and offered earnest prayers. I will never forget her shocked look as she recovered moments later and realized she hadn't died! She was dismayed and a bit embarrassed. But it was also clear she had wanted Gordon there, and he had been away at work.

I would come to call these episodes "practice runs." When one has used an old body for ninety years it is not easy to give it up. I have more than once seen the disbelief on the faces of invalids, awakening from a world of reverie or dream where they have had the feeling of freedom and movement, and then realized with a shock they are still inhabiting a crippled old body.

But Grandma made up for it. Sometimes, with a sly triumphant glance and an "I dare-you-to-say-it-isn't-so" look she would tell me, "See that tree out there? I was up there this morning," or "Well, I drove down to the post office today." She was constantly reliving themes of cooking for big gangs, something she had loved to do as much as she loved all kinds of savory food.

Mary Edna was hyper-modest about her own body. Though frontier born, it was a Victorian era she'd lived in and she well reflected the attitudes. She once reported how one scandalous lady in her home town had dared to show her ankle as she alighted from the city street car. It was a time when the fashionable grand pianos had their plump legs draped with great fringed shawls lest they be suggestive. Pregnant women were not to be seen in public so Mary Edna stayed home, cuddled up to the wood stove and ate herself up to two hundred pounds with the coming of her first child. When she was ready to deliver her twelve pound daughter, she lay in bed with covers clutched up to her chin and, while gripped in massive labor, only stared stoically at the attending doctor and never uttered a sound. He eventually realized it was up to him to discern when his services were needed.

It was therefore an event of bemused delight for all of us when, early one morning, Grandma threw off all these old restraints. I had an intercom by my bed so I could hear her awake, but this day I was slow in coming. When I entered the room, she was waiting for me stark naked, sitting up with her legs over the side, and her tiny gnarled hands furiously shaking the bed rails. Her old breasts, once round and pendulous, hung flat to her waist, and every ounce of the now wrinkled little body was telling me she wanted attention now! Hair wildly askew, her eyes black and dashed with anger, she sputtered like a little wet hen. I stifled my smiles and hopped to my duties with apologies. But such outbursts were rare.

One can often experience layers of personality peeling away in the dying process like the layers of an onion. For most of us some of the layers underneath aren't going to be all that pretty in the light of day. But with Grandma each layer underneath was as good and true as the one above. She was authentic to the core. Most often, she gave grateful sighs for the care we gave her, and for the beauty of the natural world she enjoyed from her window. She often expressed how she wished she could do more for us.

It wasn't all easy. The children loved her, but the teenagers, watching Grandma's increasing distancing and feebleness and facing the impending death while they were at their "immortal" adolescent phase of life, experienced the pain of her going. And I, as with the care of a newborn, became exhausted with the constant demands and often had to nap whenever she did. Days centered around her needs, laundry, food, hygiene and comfort. With such work, one learns we often have to go the extra mile we didn't think we could possibly go. When I counsel friends about care giving, I often call this the "last straw effect," when the depth of your commitment is tested to the full. Then things change. Hard as it was, it was also one of the most fulfilling and rewarding times in our lives. The children later told us that caring for Grandma was one of the most important experiences of their lives.

The night Grandma died, the Christian Community minister came and gave her communion and a last anointing. All the family gathered solemnly in the candlelit room. There was a majesty to the moment. With a tender gentleness the priest leaned toward her. "Grandma, this is substance to make us inclined to love," and he put the tiniest fragment of consecrated bread on her tongue and made the sign on her forehead.

She was only semi-conscious and spent the evening taking long-spaced, rasping breaths that were hard for us, especially the children, to bear. They tendered their prayers and good-byes. It was not easy. I sang for her, including one of her favorites, "Swing Low Sweet Chariot." She was putting up a long, but a sound and good, labor. Would she last the night? It was a cold, windswept moonlit night, clean and clear following winter storms. Earlier that evening we had been surprised to see a white owl flitting back and forth in the old sycamore tree Grandma had loved to watch from her window. The next day would be February 29th, leap year. It would be like her to pick such a day.

The evening wore on. My husband told me he would stay with her while I caught some sleep. Bone weary, I trudged the three flights of stairs to our bedroom in the old country home and immediately fell into deep sleep. About one in the morning, I heard the owl hooting around the house. Gordon came to the bottom of the stairs and urgently called my name. I leapt from bed, and flew down the steps, scarcely touching them. I ran into her room just in time to take her into my arms. Her eyes were wide open, she was conscious and "far seeing" into the realms beyond us, across the threshold. Gordon supported her with his powerful arms from behind, and I embraced her to complete the circle. With our last words ringing ardently around her, "Grandma, we love you!" Mary Edna left that old body and was born into the spirit. Her eyes were extraordinary to witness. The soul light, through which we shine our essence to one another, was leaving. The spark, the light of spirit presence, gradually dimmed, and just slowly faded away. She was gone. Her eyes were still wide open.

We laid her gently back on the bed, closed her eyes and placed the tiny wrinkled hands over her heart. She had made it! We sat in awe, our hearts so full and opened wide to the wonder of it all. It was totally quiet. The peace, the incredible peace! The shell of the body was empty beyond emptiness, while the atmosphere around it was full to overflowing. We sat in the dark beside the bed and basked in the sense of her triumphant expanding spirit. There was nothing to do. She no longer needed blankets or warmth or slippers or water or touch.

After a time we went up and called the sleeping children, one by one. They came downstairs into the room, now graced and holy, with reluctant wonder. The gangly teenaged son remarked, "This isn't spooky at all!" We huddled and hugged. Then we all went out on the back lawn, into the clean, chill winter night, looked up to the glittering stars and felt the sweet, cleansing wind. There was an excitement to it, a wonder for her deed of transition. We chattered and shivered and stamped our feet and talked about the wonderful owl that had come just this night. Then into the wind and the star spangled night, together we breathed our last farewell of hope, sadness, gratitude and joy for this wonderful grandmother.

I spent the rest of the night in her room. The undertaker didn't need to be called until morning. In the candlelight, I looked at her countenance, now still and quiet. I was amazed. In death the round wrinkled cheeks and chins had fallen away. The cuddly grandmother had vanished. Now was revealed the strong, high-bridged nose, the firm resolute mouth, the dignified repose. It was the countenance of a warrior. The iron character that had formed her core had risen up to the surface. It took my breath away. So this is the presence that stood behind her stoic strength and enduring moral resolve!

It was a gesture that faded slowly in the following three days. But this is something I experience again and again at birth and at death. For a time right after birth, babies can give a fleeting glimpse of their eternal personality, a glimpse of who they truly are and might become. Then, within a few hours the countenance moulds to "generic" baby, all forehead and no chin. At death, too, there can be a sweep of sculpturing power on the features which momentarily reveals the hand of the individual's spirit. It is as though the mortal clay is briefly made transparent at these mighty threshold transitions and can speak the deeper reality. Then natural forces take over or an expression is set through the embalming process.

Our eighteen-year-old son, Gary, had already made his great-grandmother's casket. During the Christmas before her passing, the family had trooped up to the third story play room where we sang Christmas carols and rubbed the casket to a warm and burnished finish with sweet-smelling oil. It was made of pine, just right for her. For the kids, the whole thing was a bit crazy and kind of wonderful all at the same time. It was their first home death. As teenagers, they were concerned with the opinions of the rest of the world. After all, other families didn't make coffins for their relatives and certainly not before they died! (Of course, this didn't keep them from gleefully playing in the casket when Gary first brought it home!) On the other hand they were proud of their contributions.

As we were preparing the casket with fragrant pine boughs in the back yard and were lining it with one of the magenta curtains that had been in her room, a teenaged son brought the question, "But what will the neighbors think?"

"They should think we really care," I replied with conviction.

We wanted her at home for three days before the funeral. This was not only to give full closure for everyone, but to hold a vigil as well.* Many community friends joined the family for the event as we read, prayed, sang and warmed her journey into spiritual existence with a stream of continuous supportive thoughts through our round-the-clock devotion. An undertaker was involved as the body needed to be shipped to Colorado where her only sister lived. He said it was the first time in sixteen years someone had wanted the body at home. I was a little concerned about how things were going for our eight-year-old son, Colin Michael, when the body came back home after being prepared at the mortuary. I asked him if everything was okay. "Oh, yes," he replied nonchalantly, "Grandma is just up in heaven looking down on her little old bones!"

For the three days, Grandma lay in honor in her little sunny, rose-tinted room by the kitchen. She had cared for people all her life, and we felt she would have chosen that role in death as well. Her home death and our honoring celebration of her life which followed it allowed over a hundred and twenty men, women and children to have their first experience with death. It was not in a hushed and somber mortuary but in the midst of a life-filled family home. In the nearby kitchen, people visited, laughed, shared coffee and the generous offerings of food that come with such occasions. Outside, the children were swinging on the rope swing and playing in the sandbox, the chickens were crowing and scratching, the teenagers were talking on the phone, and the back door was slamming with frequent comings and goings.

In a certain way it was like a royal funeral ceremony with Grandma, the queen, holding court and signaling the passing of the kingdom. People would go into her room, alone or in groups, just to be there. Children who had gone to kindergarten in that room, now ten or twelve years old, came back to sing a song, bring a precious stone, a picture, or flowers. Her room filled with cards and tributes and childish gifts. One child proudly played for Grandma on her violin, a southern mountain tune. The young visitors could satisfy their curiosity by touching her hand. Grandma was still taking care of the children.

Gratitude for the wholesomeness of the experience with Grandma was expressed by family after family as they visited in those three days. Of course, it was an intense and confronting experience for many. But it was also death as part of life, a natural part of life. Friends who came to sit alone with her for a quiet hour through the days and nights expressed their feeling of being in her spiritual presence by writing in her "book" that lay on a table nearby.

"Thank you, Grandma, for the blessing you have given, to me and to the children. Help me carry in some way the joy of your spirit and love of the children."

"As I sit here I feel the strength and peacefulness that you leave to all of us."

"I will take with me today encouragement for others that life is beautiful."

"Thank you for sharing your strength with me."

"May we always see you in the flight of the white owl, the softness, the purity, the freedom and joy. We love you dearly."

"It is my birthday. How wonderful to live with Grandma on this special day. Grandma's passing is a light in a new day and a new way. May we all be so blessed."

"Grandma has given me a special gift and continues to be an inspiration in the spiritual worlds which lie before me. Thank you, Grandma."

And eighteen-month-old Cedar, a frequent visitor and friend, did a dance around the room and sang a song of joy, "La, la, la, la, LA!".

One of the first concerns for most people is whether or not young children should have this experience. In truth, young children are still very close to the spiritual world and do not experience death as adults do. Unless there is deep fear and trauma demonstrated in the adults around them, which they can reflect, the children will usually be open and unafraid. There can be exceptions, of course, and the adults need to be sensitive to the individual child's needs.

One young mother who had never experienced a death came to honor Grandma, but she left her two-year-old son in the car behind the house while she came to briefly pay her respects. She did not want to expose the young boy to a fearful experience. She walked into the sunny room with trepidation and reverent steps.

Just as she was taking it in, the two-year-old escaped from the car and burst into the room. His mother was startled and distraught, feeling one must be quiet and holy in such a situation. Of course, the two-year-old would have none of it. He ran to the casket, grasped one of the handles and tried to rock it! The mother flushed with embarrassment, but I laughed, "It's just fine. Yes, that is Grandma's cradle. You can rock it for her," I told the child. The mother relaxed and the lively boy eagerly investigated each rock, flower, and picture in the room.

Then it was time to go. The mother lifted the child in her arms and now, for the first time, he could see into the casket. But he had no interest in the body and gave it only a cursory glance. Then looking heavenward, he addressed the spiritual presence that filled the room, as he looked with shining eyes up above the casket. With chubby fingers, he joyfully waved and repeatedly said, "Bye-bye, bye-bye." The mother was astounded, and I laughed with the sheer wonder of what I had just witnessed. "And a little child shall lead them!"

On the third day we closed the casket, sang together and took hands around it for a final farewell. Then after our solemn finalities, we found the casket wouldn't go out the door! It was too big. The only solution was to take it out those windows Grandma had so often flown through in her thoughts. We had a great laugh about it, and had no doubt Grandma had wanted some fun to be part of it all. We decorated the church with Navajo blankets, rich in design and color beneath the beautiful pine casket and brought some evergreen boughs and rocks as well, all fitting for this lady who had lived so close to mother earth. With tears, joy, songs and her life story we celebrated the ninety-three years of living on this planet by a remarkable individual.

When we returned home from the service, a rainbow was touching down right next to our back lawn in the horse pasture, something I have never seen so close before or since. It came to me that when a soul goes through the threshold gate with such special nobility that a white owl announces the passage and a large community comes to honor her, then, too, the rainbow bridge might also appear showing the way of the soul's ascent to heaven.**

*See **THE VIGIL AND THE THREE DAYS AFTER DEATH**

See **SPECIAL SIGNS IN NATURE

Grandma Mary Edna Goodman
and her great-granddaugher
Mary Edna

Grandma's 90th Birthday Celebration

Making Grandma's famous popcorn balls

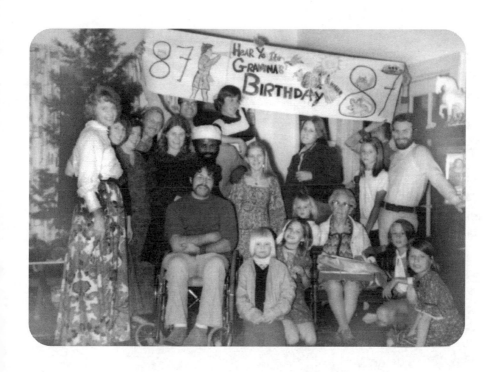

Family and Community Friends Celebrate Grandma's Birthday
and
Her Farewell Blessing Time

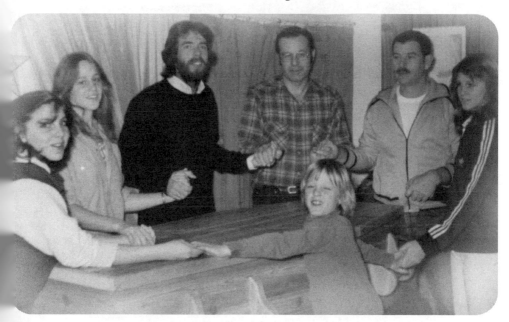

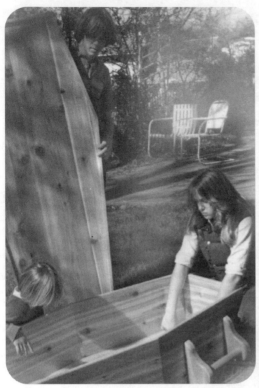

Mary Edna prepares her great-grandmother's casket with her brothers

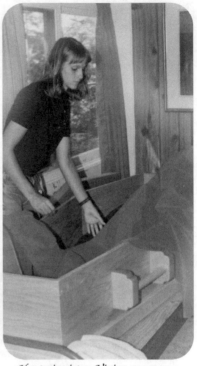

Her twin sister, Vivian prepares a casket for her grandfather

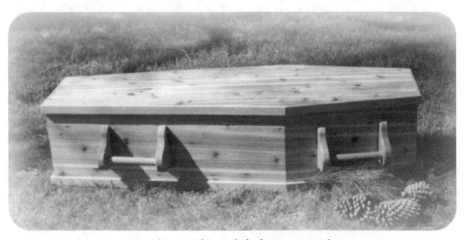

Grandma's casket made by her great-grandson, Gary

GRANDMA'S GIFTS FLOW INTO COMMUNITY LIFE

Mary Joins the Work

Of all our children, I worried the most about our sixteen-year-old Mary during the time Grandma was ending her life journey in our home. While they all adored Grandma, it was this daughter that bore her name, Mary Edna, and they were especially close. As Grandma diminished in size, in humor, in appetite, and in interactions with the family, I sometimes saw Mary turn away, her jaw clenched and pain in her eyes as she left the room.

Adolescence is an especially difficult time to have a loved one die. Young people are bursting into life with a restless vibrancy that can make them feel invincible. They are rebelling and resisting the older generations to come into their own era and their own individuality. In the ordinary scheme of things the adults are supposed to be there for them; to admire, to encourage, to be shocked, to show off for, and to be an immovable and predictable anchor to give firmness and resistance as they hammer out their new strength and selfhood. It can seem unfair and out of season when the adult leaves the field and dies.

During the time of Grandma's dying, I realized Mary was finding excuses not to be at home. She was working after school driving a delivery truck for a spa company and she began signing up for delivery runs to other states that would take her away all weekend. Yet when she was home, no one could have been more attentive to Grandma. I often found them sitting together, Mary with her arm around her great-grandmother's shoulder as she whispered their little jokes and encouraged Grandma's famous giggle. She would take her outdoors for some fresh air, carefully tucking a soft, woolen robe over her lap to make sure she was warm enough and once outside, she would find a colorful blossom to drop in her lap or bring the dog close to cheer her. At meals she selected the most tasty and tender morsels of food for Grandma and often fed them to her as well. I watched it all but said little knowing Mary, like everyone involved in this coming transition, had to find her own way to work with it.

The night Grandma died, with long wracking rattles of breath, it was almost too much. Mary was there with all the family for the last rites. She pledged her love to her beloved grandparent and then left the room along with the other children who were each suffering in their own way. Yet after

27

the death, Mary would let no one else do the final preparation work to make the casket beautiful.

The most unforgettable moment for me happened on the third day after Grandma's death. It was time to close the casket. Knowing Mary's special connection to her great-grandmother, her father and I had agreed on a gift for her. We took her with us into the room where Grandma lay surrounded by the scent of beeswax candles and bright fragrant flowers. As we stood beside the casket, Gordon reached for the tiny, life-worn hand of his grandmother and removed her golden wedding band.

Our daughter stood between us, ramrod straight, at once vulnerable and strong in her youthful beauty. Her face, framed by her long brown hair, was expectant, solemn and deeply intent. Gordon and I both offered a few words about this special moment. Then we watched as this young girl-becoming-woman slowly reached out her hand and with the greatest reverence, received the golden ring. It was a moment of initiation at the threshold of death—like a noble youth receiving knighthood.

So was passed the legacy of love, hope and years of a life honorable met, down across the generations. From that day on, Mary Edna, the younger, wore the golden ring. She has worn it through her life, a constant and treasured symbol of her grandmother's love.

Yet despite the fulfillment of this moment in our lives, for a long time after Grandma's passing I would sometimes worry that the home deaths had been too hard on the family, especially Mary. I knew that our expectation that our adolescents embrace the larger community during Grandma's vigil was certainly a big one for them. They felt protective of her, like she belonged just to us, and at times they expressed doubts that all these people coming to the house could really know how special she was. The threshold of death stretches us all in ways we may not want to go.

Though I knew in my heart every decision we made then was a truthful one, the nagging doubt remained. I wondered how it would turn out for them in the long run. Then three years later, when she entered college, Mary wrote a paper, which was later graded with an "A" on "Why Families Should Bring Their Loved Ones Home to Die." I gave a sigh of relief.

Several years after Grandma made her transition, my godson died. His family was among the many friends that supported us so generously through the grandparents' deaths. He was a beautiful boy with golden curls and a wonderful face. He had a disease that became increasingly difficult to endure and eventually he was confined to a wheelchair. He was considered a miracle child even at a young age, but with the selfless care of his family, and the strength of his remarkable spirit, he lived many years longer than might have been expected. The stoic courage with which he faced the pain, along with the radiating, uplifting goodness he bestowed on everyone he met, brought him many admirers. In his brief life, he inspired a vast community of friends both young and old all across the country. When he died suddenly at twelve, countless people felt the loss.

I was to care for his body. Mary volunteered to help me. Knowing how hard Grandma's passing had been for her, I assured her she didn't need to feel she had to take part. But it was the very gift of her great-grandmother's death that gave her the experience and resolve to be part of this one. She had loved the boy and she wanted to show it with care. They had a special connection for, in what was to be his last month of life, she had been at his home every day remodeling the family's kitchen. They had shared a special camaraderie in those days around jokes and music they both enjoyed.

His body was brought from the hospital to a mortuary. There Mary and I worked together in a dreary, windowless room, gently bathing and dressing his dear form, so long and lovingly attended by his parents and now laid, still and quiet, on a marble slab. Even that morning his parents had bathed and prepared him, for they expected to have school pictures taken that day. In the end, with his gentle and devoted mother beside him, he had died in his father's arms, even as he been received into his father's hands when he was born. Mary was filled with awe and reverence. We marveled at how his great spirit had been able to endure the trials of physical life for as long as it had. We both felt the honor and privilege, as godmother, as friend, to be his last caregivers.

We placed the body in a casket our family had made, put it in Mary's pickup truck and drove to the family's home in the foothills. The parents wanted the vigil to be in the workshop of the barn. There would be multitudes of friends coming for him, including many, many children, as well as adults, for he was a friend to them all. We made everything as beautiful and right as we could.

Years before, I had attended the funeral of a twelve-year-old child, and had been incensed that the funeral company had covered the honest, raw earth from her grave with plastic artificial grass. By contrast, there was such an authenticity about this setting-the work bench with the carpenter tools he and his brothers had so enthusiastically used to make knightly swords and countless other projects, and his favorite baseball shirt laid out along with photos and offerings.

Our threshold work completed, Mary and I drove home. It had been an intense and fulfilling day for us. Both of us were partly across the threshold ourselves, having been deeply engaged in the mystery of death and the wonder of the timeless, while simultaneously working at a task that needed to be completed in an earthbound time frame. Mary put the last tape of music the boy had given her in the tape deck and, as we drove, the melody washed over us and tears streamed unabated down our faces. She told me of their special connection and we agreed on how wonderful it had been to know him.

Then it followed that I was able to share with this daughter, as never before with my family, the deep place in me from which I receive a calling for this work. I told her how I felt each human life is unique, that no biography is the same, and every life is a sacred story of the individual's spirit quest and mission in life. The setting of the final act, I felt, should be as artistic and beautiful as we can humanly make it for the hallowed work of closure and farewells. Above all, we would give honor to that singular journey of human endeavor, and our caring support to the beginning of the person's next experience in spiritual existence.

She understood. As mother and daughter, now co-workers, we had just fulfilled that role together. When we parted we held each other a long time and wept and were never closer.

Shauna

Shauna lived with us for nearly two years. She was an elementary school teacher in her mid-thirties, and we had many common interests, but it was the dog that brought her to our home. When no landlords would take him when she was trying to find a place to rent, she settled on a tiny room in the old water tower behind our house rather than be separated from her beloved canine companion.

Bespeaking her Scandanavian heritage, she was tall, lithe and fair. Her fine spun blonde hair hung half way down her back. Chutney, the little black dog, adored her, and as they took up residence in the second story of the water tower we called her Rapunzel.

Shauna had never been close to a death in her life. At our home she would experience two deaths that ultimately brought new dimensions to her being and brought her, through suffering, to a place where she could help others along the way. The first was Chutney's death.

The little dog was handsome and curly, but darned independent. One day Gordon and I took a walk down the street and Chutney dashed to follow us. We tried to order him back to the house, but he ignored us and trotted with resolute purpose up the hill and into an oncoming car. The fatal thud sounded and brought death instantaneously. Full of sadness, we carried the limp body back to the house and the back yard.

Gordon went to tell Shauna. She was near hysteria with the shock, and inconsolable with grief. Meanwhile, I took the little dog, washed away the blood and laid him on a board. I moved the body to a natural position and smoothed the soft, silky black hair so the sight would not be so overwhelming. Then, after a while, I went to Shauna and quietly told her it would be important for her to come and see him.

She didn't want to. It was too painful, too fresh, too awful. I urged her to try; it would be important for both of them. At last she came. The sight of her dear companion lying still in death brought a fresh spasm of grief. Sorrow washed over both of us, and the tears flowed. Then after a time, she was able to reach gingerly toward the little form and stroke him, slowly finding her center inwardly to make decisions about where to bury him and how to complete the process. She was deeply human in her sorrow, radiantly beautiful in her courage to ultimately face the death and find some closure in the reality of the situation. Both are deeply important aspects of dealing with this threshold.

31

Shauna had loved Grandma Mary Edna, too. They had often spent time together and enjoyed one another's company. When she came home after Grandma's death, she had real trepidation about seeing the body. It took her several tries before she could enter the room. We didn't pressure her. Finally the moment came when she could stand before the mystery of human death. Her tender heart and big soul encompassed it deeply.

Shauna helped us through the next days in preparing for the funeral in every way she could. One could almost sense her grounding, centering and growing throughout the process. She found solace and a rightness in how we were dealing with the death. It would be a prophetic time.

Less than a year later, a colleague in her school died suddenly. It was Shauna that was called upon, and who took the responsibility to direct the process of bringing the body back to the family home and helping in the preparation of a community vigil and celebration. She called me on the phone to consult on the details, and I was impressed with the timbre of confidence in her voice. She was ready for the task; she had been prepared. The grateful widow and community were inspired by her leadership in helping to create a natural harmony, rightness and beauty around the poignant event.

To say I was incredibly proud of her would be an understatement. To be sure, I gave thanks to dear Grandma Mary Edna and the beloved little dog, Chutney, who had both given her the deeper and greater soul capacities to carry the gift to another community.

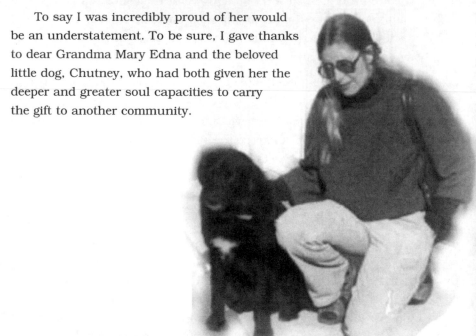

See **TOWARD NEW COMMUNITY**   *Chutney & Shauna*

MY TEACHER

A friend told me I must share this story. I had not intended to do so, but I sense she was right. The events were so fundamental to shaping who I would later become and to inspiring my threshold work.

The summer I turned fourteen, I had a significant inner experience. It is hard to describe—probably a kind of "rite of passage" within the soul comes the closest. It was an awakening to a prophetic awareness of my own destiny.

My parents had a wonderful mountain home, theirs for over fifty years, where the family spent the summers. I first learned to walk there among the pine trees and the golden scents of summer. Something about first standing upright in three-dimensional space and mastering my own toddler body there must have given me a deep and joyful connection to everything in that land and all that could awaken me to the world. When I was eight, I would climb the tall pine trees to the tip top and cling to the swaying trunk with grubby, pitch covered fingers, rejoicing in my sense of all-seeing omnipotence and feeling the wind in my face.

The cabin my father built had no electricity, no running water and only an outdoor privy. He dug a cistern and built a system of gutters and pipes to collect the rain water as it ran off the roof of the cabin. Pumping a squeaky, long handled pump, we pulled the precious substance up from the depths and collected it in galvanized buckets. One room had a fireplace. There were big meadows, trees, quiet, horses, freedom and stars. It was a child's paradise.

We made improvements to the cabin gradually as time and money from my father's teaching salary permitted. One summer, we made the front porch. We poured concrete around bronze colored stones of gold bearing quartz which had come from the old gold mines that had thrived on the ranch in the nineteenth century. Named the Gold King, Queen and Jack, the mines would later give the ranch its name, the K & Q. We children helped to build the porch, including my brother who was going off to war. Hauling and turning, tugging and fitting, we worked the jagged stones into the most artistic positions and then set them in the cement which we mixed with a long hoe in a great, flat hopper. It was important and beautiful work. We were empowered with our creative deed, and I now think of the wisdom of my teacher/father to bring this solid family creation just then in the face of the son leaving for an unknown future in the war. We were all proud of the results.

Facing south, the porch warmed in the summer sun. Yet there was usually a cool and soothing breeze sighing through the nearby pines. I loved to lie on its sun baked surface, warmed from above and below and dream the stuff of a young girl's dreams. It was there the vision-prophecy-knowing came. On a still afternoon, as I lay basking in quiet and the sun of a beautiful day, I knew, "I will have six children." There was a flood of joyful soul response. Yes! Then, as if that thought triggered some inward resolve in response, it went further: "I want to drink the full cup of life . . . and I want to meet many, many interesting people." The mantle of my coming destiny rested warm and hopeful about me that afternoon. I held it in my heart and told no one. It would all come true. But the journey from the dream of that lovely day to reality would be fraught with lessons for the soul and forged in the fire.

When the wonderful husband came into my life, we began our journey together bravely, pretty much in total poverty and quite confident of our ability to take life on. We both had jobs: he was in his final apprenticeship year to become a pharmacist and was paid sub-living wages. I was secretary for the County Agriculture agent.

Years of hard work in college began to take a toll on my health. I had held jobs long hours and carried a full course load, but still could not resist the many other extracurricular sports and social life. My thyroid had been compromised, and the longed-for children didn't come, or they came ever so briefly and slipped away. Finally a doctor identified the problem. Now surely everything would be all right. But it wasn't.

How young and vulnerable and full of trembling hope I was! Aching with longing for a child and trying to be sensible as each month unfolded, I was alternately swept with hope and fear. The pregnancies came, and with each one I not only hoped, but my body hoped also—the missed period, the tender swelling breasts, each cell marshaled in readiness to receive the child. Two months passed and then another disappointment. I was again "unchosen." Then I was pregnant again. Surely this would be the time. During this pregnancy, my husband's father died tragically in a plane crash when I was two months along. As we went through the shock and sorrow, I was resolved this child should come into the family to help honor the grandfather's legacy of life. But it was not to be. At three-and-a-half months, the contractions began. I lay in bed willing with every ounce of my being for them to stop, but they moved relentlessly on.

"Not now," I pleaded, "not with Gordon's father just crossing over." Praying and weeping, I lay suspended between desperate hope and the reality of this world.

A golden light filled the room. It was very bright. The message permeated and enveloped me, "All will be well." I clung to the blessing and desperately hoped it meant now. But the tide swept on. I rose awkwardly, cramping and bleeding profusely as I miscarried and my husband aided me. We grabbed towels and struggled to the car and went to the hospital. Anesthetic, curettage, all matter-of-fact, and condolences afterward, "You can try again," we were told.

I was experienced now and tougher. But why had the message come that everything would be all right? There wasn't a place to talk about it, so I didn't. I worked. I made a home. I had learned that life is not always fair and it can be hard. All around me women produced babies, some wanted, some not wanted. Most of them took it all casually, as a matter of course, while I sat on the sidelines.

My husband's widowed mother moved to town. My father and I helped design and supervise the building of the home she wanted, a small consolation in her loss. The home was lovely, and she was pleased. During the next year, I became pregnant again. This time I would do everything in my power to see that it worked. I was going to bed. My mother-in-law kindly took us in. Seasoned with seven children, one of whom had died at four, she must have thought our measures extreme. However, she was solicitous and respectful of our space and prepared meals for us along with her family. I only got up briefly, careful not to do any activity that would start the contractions. I can't remember what all I did as I lay in bed. I must have read and slept a lot. I did not make baby clothes. Most surely I counted the days, marking the calendar as each day was accomplished and rising weakly each month for doctor's appointments. Five, six months passed; it appeared to be working! I was up now and could do more. The child would be viable now! The doctor gave us the go ahead to try living on our own.

We looked eagerly for a rental house, not an apartment. It had to be a house; it could be very small, but a real house. We were going to be a family. A family! We needed room for a baby to play and grow up with earth and cats and a dog. Never mind that the house we found had awful, dark green living room walls. We could fix that, and we did. Out came the paint brushes and rollers. The kitchen needed curtains, but I could make those. Best of all, there was a small second bedroom, the holy of holies, a baby's room. We had *our* castle. What love we lavished there! Pink or blue wouldn't do for the walls—it had to be a soft peach to delight anyone's eye. I found a quilt-like fabric patterned with pink and blue to cover an ancient family rocker and trim the curtains. The nesting instincts were burgeoning with pent-up creativity, held back by all those early anxious months. I loved to sew and particularly enjoyed designing stylish western clothes. I made a pretty peasant-style dress with tiered skirts, carefully sewing in snaps for a concealed opening in the front so I could nurse my baby. I was young and confident I would recover my shape quickly. I could be fashionable *and* a nursing mother as well. I never felt happier.

As soon as we moved in, I began a garden. There had to be a garden. The earth was rich and dark. I had noted this before renting the place. I couldn't wait to get my hands in the soil. I relished pulling weeds from spades full of dirt. Mother earth, dark rich and fecund, like me, and I like Her. I was home.

I gathered seed packets in reverent rituals. "How wonderful is seed-packet art!" I thought. Crimson radishes, the crisp white and verdant hues of green onions, the plump orange of perfect carrots, all promised the fruit-ful wonder of what is hidden in the tiny seeds rattling in their packages. And I, like them, was carrying the magic seed of a coming child. People wonder why the Mona Lisa has her smile. Dear friends, surely she was pregnant! The quiet mystery, the great secret of being pregnant before it is told; to be the chalice, the vessel bearing the great and holy jewel of new life, the deepest woman mystery.

I was given a baby shower. Big and awkward, I basked in the attention with shy joy. I was joining the multitudes, joining the great ranks of motherhood. The patter, the giggles, the chattering and gentle natterings of the women, preparing delicacies, holding up tiny garments and exclaiming over the preciousness, the colors, the texture, all swirled around me, blessing me like the beams of summer sun that had foretold my future. I rode home like a queen and tucked my little stash of garments away in drawers and shelves, fingering each one or holding it to my cheek as I did so. All was well.

But all was not well. I was not quite eight months along. The doctor had a premonition of problems and sent me to a specialist. Crisp, dark and effi-

cient, the doctor ordered X-rays. Through the awkward movements of climbing on the cold X-ray table, I trembled with trepidation. The doctor called us
in for the results. Clipped on the wall the film hung showing the outline of a
large baby, strong in body, with well-formed limbs, hands and feet. But, as
the physician explained with professional proficiency, the head was not
developed enough. The skull was not fully formed. It was an anencephalic
baby with the head about half the size it would normally be. The black and
gray of the X-rays swam before my eyes. The doctor went on as kindly as he
could manage. The baby would die at birth. With an underdeveloped nervous system, it would not have the ability to live outside the womb. We were
young and this would soon be over and we could try again. He left the room.

In that five minutes, my life spun chaotically out of control, out of any
control I had of it. All my careful plans to evade problems with bed rest were
for naught. I carried a child who could not have survived in any event. With
the shock, time seemed to stop long enough for the moment to sear a lasting imprint inwardly as I clung to a fragile point of consciousness. Then the
surrounding world blurred and became surreal.

Gordon was magnificent. He offered no recriminations, no regrets, only
deep and patient support. I knew it was a huge disappointment for him, following right on the loss of his father, but he rallied to my needs when he was
not working his long hours.

We returned to a house, once so filled with life and hope, now gray, cold
and soulless. Curtains seemed to hang limp at the windows, The garden, so
lovingly begun, where I might have healed a bit, reeked with the desecration
of the neighborhood cats. I gave up. I couldn't wait to move away.

The doctor did not want to start labor. I had five weeks to go. In those
days, obstetricians did not do vaginal births after cesarean sections and he
did not want to resort to this as they also did not do repeated C-sections.
This procedure would limit the children I might be able to have. We all agreed
we would wait.

So began my purgatory on earth. The child was alive. It kicked and
pushed at my sides, especially at night as I lay staring into the darkness as
my husband rested softly beside me. I was a vessel for life and a vessel for
death. Like some strange blonde Western Kali, the Hindu mother Goddess of
destruction, the destroyer of life, the giver of life, I bore life and death within
my womb at once. This moving child under my heart would die.

How could I connect with the anomaly that was my child? I could not hate this being, yet I did not have the depth of spiritual awareness then to encompass it all. But the experience would surely shape me toward a path of spiritual longing. I mustered all the love I could manage for the strange, hapless being within me, but all was intertwined with my benumbed suffering. We had few friends in that town where we had recently moved, so we told virtually no one. Those whom we did tell expressed sympathy but stayed away. They didn't know what to say. An abnormal child was an unfathomable and nearly unspeakable disappointment to everyone. I did not seek company. Each day was a living hell. My mother was gone during these months. My father stood helplessly by, the pain of my trials written on his face, sadness in his eyes and a tightness in his jaw. He was caught in the frustration that there was nothing he could do to make it better for his daughter.

I dismantled the baby's room. Between bouts of weeping, each garment was coolly and efficiently folded, taped away in a box and put high on a shelf. We removed the rocker and stripped the room. It had no purpose anymore.

After five interminable weeks the labor began at last. At the first sign, the doctor immediately took action and added drugs to expedite the process. He clearly felt compassion for me in my dull and wretched endurance of the ordeal. After a rough delivery, I was moved away from the maternity ward so I wouldn't have to painfully watch the other mothers with their newborn infants. I lay stunned and torn asunder from the harsh birth, for the small head could not prepare the way as in a usual birth. I lay sleepless through the night staring into nothing. After midnight, they brought a woman and put her in the room with me. She had aborted herself.

"Why, dear God?" I asked. I had longed so greatly for a child and now in this hour of despair, how was I to shape some sort of a relationship to this woman who had done away with her own baby? She was not bright and drawled in rough language of her ordeal. She wondered at the amount of her bleeding, complained of her cramps, and repeatedly called for more attention from the nurses. Absorbed as she was in her event, I don't recall if she asked about mine. If so, I did not answer in detail. It was a strange test. Would I later be able to form some kind of compassion for her and the desperation that had led her to her act? I could hardly do so then.

My milk came in. The body did not know the child had died. It prepares no matter what. I spoke to the doctor to see if I could give milk for a needy child. Wisely he talked me out of what would have been a long laborious process of breast pumping. Surely there was something in all of this that could serve; surely there was some need for it, something to give the world? We gave the little body to a medical school for research. It was a decision I don't believe I would make now, but our longing for some good to come in the wake of it all was very great.

Afterward I was shattered for some time. My confidence was utterly shaken. I was not a mother, and perhaps would never be one. I was like a house felled in an earthquake that had to be rebuilt brick by brick to realize who I was to be. I worked. I struggled to heal. Two years later, I became pregnant again. I had no shower, made no baby clothes and did not dare to hope. The nine-and-a-half pound baby girl who came to fulfill the prophecy restored our shaken faith, and we began our parenting, which would indeed include six children.

Not very many years later, I would look back on this event as a pivotal one in my whole life. Because of it, my husband and I never resented the incredible demands and needs of our family. We know how precious life is, and we were only too willing to care for our children. We were deeply grateful to be parents. But the spirit of this first child, ah, what a teacher! In retrospect, I have only the profoundest gratitude for the gift of this child, who took me to the depths of my being so I could slowly but surely begin to find God and life again. This being, who could not see the light of day, has been the most incredible source of light in my life and lives behind every ideal I strive for to bring aid to others. This child, my spiritual connection to a higher source, is a hidden force behind my resolve to support children and parents, my work for humane home births wherever possible, and the spirit-filled ways to work with death and dying. This child, my teacher, allowed me to hold under my heart simultaneously the great mystery of life and the great mystery of death in one powerful, life-changing experience.

See **OUR CONNECTIONS TO THOSE WHO HAVE DIED**

A CHILD NAMED EMBER HOPE

Decades later, a touching epilogue to this story was inscribed into my life by the wonderful parents of a child called Ember Hope. Gail, the mother, and I had met only briefly before Ember came. We had connected a few times over our mutual concerns for healthy parenting and children's education. But, on this occasion, she called me to tell me she was pregnant with her third child, and it was not going well. She wanted to talk about her options around the situation.

I welcomed her into our home. She was advanced in pregnancy and the lines around her eyes showed her strain and fatigue. Her face had a gentle, noble demeanor. Her whole being expressed soul nurturing capacities, an embodiment of mother giving. Even now, as she faced the death of her child, she was filled with concern to do what would be the best for this child and her family.

The house was quiet and we sat in big, blue leather chairs before a glowing fire. She told me her story in a soft voice. Tears sometimes welled in her eyes and in mine. I was touched to the core. Her child had the same syndrome as our first born, a living child that would die. Only here, before me now was a woman, who, along with her husband, was ready to honor and share this experience with family and friends. They were birthing a child that would die and were willing and open to find the ways and community support embrace the event. In the era when my husband and I went through this, one hardly talked about such a birth. We didn't know how. Certainly at that time we could hardly have found a community to support and honor all concerned.

Coming of age in the sixties, in all the good ways, Gail and her partner, George, had never lost their idealism. But even though the cultural climate now is more open to the choices they intended to make around their child's crossing, they were still pioneers in this approach. The friends and family who would gather around them had never experienced a death with a vigil at home. The couple was resolved to bring new social ritual and experience to a whole community through honoring life and staying in the flow of universal being.

I shared with Gail the story of our firstborn as our great teacher, and it helped give her hope and perspective for the trials ahead. We talked of having the baby brought home, making a cradle, having a vigil and sharing it all with her older boys, five and eight. As she debated home or hospital birth (she had good support available with either choice) I emphasized the importance of her care, her strength and recovery as she was central to everyone's well being. As we discussed each aspect of the process, she saw that her plan could be realized. I felt her sense of resolve and relief. Before she left, I knelt beside her and we prayed with our hands touching across her great, warm belly, blessing and thanking the precious child therein for its gifts to all the family and community.

Then as we looked into the glowing embers of the fire place, Gail confided brightly. "We've given the child a name...Ember Hope." My heart turned with the sounding of the name. I knew it was a girl, though Gail told me later she didn't know that for sure until the birth.

We kept in touch. They sent out announcements to family and friends inviting them to a "blessing way" ceremony for the birth three weeks later. But before it could happen, Gail went into labor and the day the blessing had been planned turned out to be the vigil day. Ember Hope was born weighing just less than five pounds, with sweet delicate features, perfect in every way but for the tiny back of her head which they covered with a silken cap. They dressed her in a beautiful gown and put her in a wooden cradle made by her father.

Gail called me the next morning and told me of the birth and the planned events. As she spoke, an incredible presence filled the space. A spirit-knowing flooded the exchange between us as I told her that this child, Ember Hope, embodies in her name everything that is asked of us as individuals of our time. First, we must face the threshold of death and strive for knowledge that the spirit transcends physical existence, and then we must act out of that faith to bring our knowing into real practical life. Secondly, we must have the fire of the spirit, the fiery resolve to commit ourselves to bringing hope and peace into our lives and the lives of others around us despite our personal struggles. Fire and Peace—what a combination! The ember of spirit warmth and light in our hearts, and hope in our actions. Ember Hope.

They brought Ember Hope home from the hospital in the cradle. Her grandmother and older brothers held her. Then they put the little cradle with the tiny child, surrounded by roses, into the crib, which was decorated with beautiful soft rainbow silk. The bedroom was lovely. As visitors came, Gail was in the living room in the big rocking chair to greet them. Nearby on a large coffee table were baskets of crayons and colored pencils and papers so anyone could draw pictures and write offerings. Many did. The kitchen overflowed with food. The children were in and out, playing in the yard.

Some visitors hesitated to go back to the bedroom. In the end, George told how he was there to embrace each one. Some would sit quietly, sing, play the guitar, or read the Bible or a children's story. "I was a little like a proud father," George later told me, "reciting her weight and birthday."

"It could have been a little better organized, maybe," he said later. "I wanted it to go well for Gail, and maybe it could have been a little more somber," he confided, "It was joyous in the living room, and the kids were in and out, downing all the food." It was clear the older brothers relished the special social activity of the day.

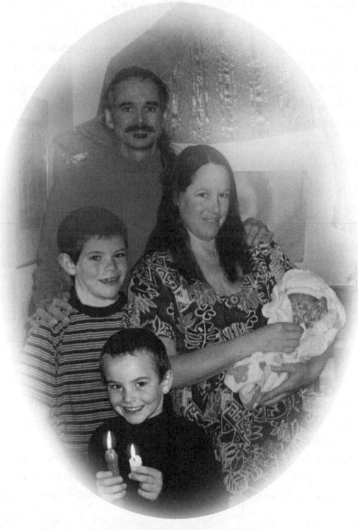

The father went on to tell me how they had gathered around the crib and sung "Amazing Grace" and "Swing Low, Sweet Chariot." Then they read a lovely children's book, *When The Sun Rose*, which brought just the right touch to the ritual. Both parents recognized that it took courage for friends and family to come, but they all did. George told me, "They were here for us and in the end, the timing was perfect. We were acting out of the sacredness of the moment....we have no doubt of that now." As he closed he told me, "I just feel happy. I slept happy. It's been a happy day."

Determined to bring consciousness and gratitude to every aspect of the process, George and Gail continued the ritual and accompanied the little body to the crematorium. Just a few decades ago, it was often considered protocol for the mother or widow to stay confined at home while others took care of the burial. A brave new world is being forged by parents like these.

I had told Gail to watch for signs in nature around the event of the birth and transition, especially birds. She had reported that the day after the birth and during the vigil, a beautiful hawk had swooped into the yard where her two sons and a friend were playing and almost took her son's cap off! The boys ran and told Gail's father and together they watched two hawks circling the house several times. After that, her son, Clarke, was followed by a hawk a number of times on his way to school.

A few months after the birth, Gail attended an art class where they were asked to paint a madonna. Gail's painting turned out to be a beautiful, open faced, golden haired mother dressed in vibrant red, looking upward, and releasing a golden brown bird to fly free.

The stories of Ember's ministry continue. Gail told me of a woman at her son's school who told her own father the story of Ember Hope. The woman had a brother who had died before she was born, but the father had never spoken about the child. With Ember's story his tears came, along with the story of her brother. The father had never cried before and now father and daughter found a new bond of caring.

Gail's own father had always been quiet and stoic in the face of death. But with Ember Hope's transition he left Gail a note, his touching tribute to his grandchild and his courageous daughter:

> "This I will remember: I walked through the door into the bed-
> room. To the left was a crib. Next to the crib was a small round table
> holding three candles—a tall one, a middle-sized one and a short

43

one. In the crib was a tiny, newly born baby girl. A beautiful little baby girl with well formed arms, hands, legs, feet and a sweet little smiling face. Only one thing was missing—life. This beautiful little baby girl was born without life. Standing next to the crib was my daughter. Her face did not show anger or bitterness. She looked as though she was saying thanks to God for letting her have a few moments with the little baby girl."*

Gail tells me that she and her father can now discuss death and birth much more easily. She knows this will make a difference with the transition of the family elders, the great grandparents.

I feel a deep gratitude to this family. Through their deed, I have vicariously had further closure for our firstborn. The shared experience has helped us all recognize the greater consciousness we have gained through the simultaneous birth and death of a child.

George and Gail have no doubt that Ember Hope is a special spirit guardian for all their family. Her story was included in their Christmas letter, and her spiritual presence continues to give a special quality to their lives. These parents exemplify the deepening spiritual strength which lives in those who can bring honor and gratitude to every aspect of life, and which gives rightness, hope and abiding peace to our experiences on earth.

See **GRIEF**

A SPIRITUAL VIEW OF DYING
I

Most people have a sense of their unique spiritual individualities and many hold the belief the human being has a higher and immortal nature as well as a temporal one. These sections throughout the book that are written in italics are for those who wish to consider the deeper spiritual aspects of death and dying. The thoughts expressed have come from many years of study, including views from ancient cultures, hours of conversation with theologians, life experience, and, above all, the study of the work of Rudolf Steiner, who had capacities to perceive spiritual realities beyond the physical phenomena. He wrote and lectured extensively from those insights. They have inspired practical healing work in all fields from education, medicine, agriculture, and work with the handicapped, to art, music, architecture, and more. In the stories presented, I have endeavored to point to incidents and statements where the activity of the spirit may be discernible in the unfolding events around preparation for death, the process of dying and the transition after death. Obviously, these chapters are only brief, initial presentations of very complex aspects of human life and death. For those interested in further research on the subjects, an extensive bibliography is offered at the end of the book.

THE VIGIL AND THE THREE DAYS AFTER DEATH

The three days after death are a special time. In any death, the people around are changed. They are changed with sympathy, grief, shock, or relief for the loved one's release from suffering in a damaged or aged body. They can be altered from every day casualness to a new sincerity of being. We are brought closer to the spiritual world by a loved one's death for it brings life near and makes it precious.

One could ask, "Why is it helpful to have the body present after death, and why read for the one who has died?" First, a basic and healthy response in those viewing the body is the immediate realization that the person they knew and loved is no longer in that body. This direct experience helps give finality and closure. Second, even though the spirit of the one who has just died can immediately touch the lives of loved ones at far distances, there is a vitality, a soul and spirit essence which remains near the body for about three days. Sitting nearby, quietly and openly, one can often feel a peace, a sense of spiritual presence, and an enhanced state of awareness.

Reading for the dead is really not all that unusual when we think it through. After all, it is customary to say prayers for them. Most people feel the validity of the special, touching connections across the threshold that are continued when the surviving spouse of a long marriage still talks, on a daily basis, to his or her loved one in the spiritual world. Reading is merely a next step that can send eternal spiritual thoughts and concepts to the individual who has crossed over, to create a surrounding ambience for their transition. This can aid in quickening the awareness of the one that has died for the process in the spiritual world.

The point of an all day and night vigil (when it is practical and reasonable to do) with readings, poetry, music and prayer, is the creation of a continuous stream of human consciousness and caring; this stream will follow the one who has made the transition. It creates an accompaniment of warmth and spirit truthfulness for the individual adjusting to a new state of existence. Spiritual substance is built up through the natural comings and goings of the family around a death, and through the prayers and readings (which can also take place far away). Such substance can be especially tangible in the close proximity of the one who has died. Those on this side are offering up gratitude, love, devotion, human warmth, and the tenderness of human sorrowing in missing the one who has crossed. The expanding soul and spirit gives back vitality and blessing which can be full of universal wisdom. The spiritual substance in the space between becomes a mutual creation. Friends in our community who come to this type of vigil for the first time often enter the room with some trepidation. Most come away amazed by the uplifting and soul altering space they have experienced there. They can feel something of the eternal, a peace and a blessing. The experience for many people during these three days can be a sense of living in an altered and elevated timeless state, though it may also be wrought with intense pain and loss.

Family members are benefited by being encouraged to do everything they feel they can or want to do around the death to create the setting and ceremony. When it is appropriate for them, family members who are able to move out of passivity in face of the experience, and put forth their will to meet it, even in small ways, make important first steps toward healing. When we can do this, we start to incorporate the event into our biography through our own initiative. The caring for the body can be a deeply fulfilling experience. Family members can also make phone calls, arrange flowers, find photos of the loved one's life to display for those who come, and make a guest book. These activities will seem natural to do. These are first steps in healing that may be more easily realized when the body is present. Sometimes when it is not, the death can seem un-real.

Common sense needs to be part of any decisions about the vigil. Family members may be exhausted from their exertions to be there for the loved one's dying process. Their sleep and recovery are priorities. Hopefully, food and help to look after children will be forthcoming. The family often has to make last minute funeral arrangements and decisions and needs to inform and meet relatives coming in for the funeral. It is obvious that friends and helpers need to be present to help schedule people to come and give support to make a full three day vigil possible. But in any situation, it is helpful if there can be a quiet period of time just after the death before the mortuary is called. This can be a time from which everyone can benefit.

During the three days after death, the one who has died is experiencing a vivid picture tableau of the life just lived. Whether the body is at home or not, as family and friends gather, the memories, the jokes, the shared stories that naturally take place at a death and the funeral become a natural support to this process. As the stories and characterizations are gathered together, they build up a picture of the individual's life. It is a wonderful spiritual support for the loved one now in the spiritual world, if some of those present are listening carefully to pick up the larger themes of the person's life. They can listen with intention to gain a deeper understanding of the spiritual biography. They can note what age the person was when life changing events occurred; what were the great challenges, both inward and outward, the special meetings and opportunities, illnesses and relationships, the cultural milieu. New appreciation and awareness can be possible now for us to develop a sense of the skein of destiny through which the individual's deeper spiritual mission tried to manifest. It is then a beautiful gift if, at the funeral ceremony, along with outer achievements, a picture of the individual's life, with the major challenges and triumphs, and a truthful picture of what that person experienced and transformed and gave back as gifts into the lives of others can shine through the eulogy.

It is always helpful for those who have passed on, as well as those remaining, when gratitude for their presence in our lives is expressed. Hopefully, whatever ritual, service or sharing that takes place around the death will reflect the solemn and powerful aspects of being a unique spiritual human being who goes through life and death on earth, and who can continue to evolve in the spiritual world while still caring for loved ones that remain here.

GRIEF

There are many good books covering the vast subject of grieving, and this book does not attempt to do so. However, the following thoughts may be helpful with regard to the connections with our loved ones who have gone on.

Grief is a tremendous and important part of human life. It must be recognized, honored, and worked through if we are to be whole human beings. Grief needs its time and its place. This powerful, transforming and deepening human emotion comes over us like waves, receding and then rising up, again and again, with over-whelming power. The great burden of grief does not come to meet us only once, but must be lifted and sifted, again and again. The hope is that each time the task is met, more healing and understanding rewards the courage to go through the process. Gradually the burden becomes more bearable through our work of trans-formation and through reaching out to others with deepened humanity.

I have felt the depths of grief to be like falling into the stars, falling into vast, dark and seemingly endless space, and never knowing if a caring presence, spiri-tually, or on this plane, will be there to hold me. Yet, in retrospect, I awakened to the realization that something that can hardly be named is, ultimately, always there with love.

The little child, dying young and innocent, has little earthly biography to add to its spiritual mission, but the power of the mission can radiate into countless lives. The tender poignancy of the child's death will always accompany the parents. However, unremitting and unending grief, especially over the death of our elders, can be paralyzing over time. It binds us into ourselves, and, when we are so pre-occupied, we are walled off from life and others. We are also cut off from our loved ones across the threshold, who cannot bridge an emotional wall that has few open-ing spaces of warmth, love and gratitude where they might enter.

Our loved ones need to be recognized as spiritual creators in their own jour-ney. This may be very hard to understand, for, from an earthly perspective, the tim-ing and setting of some deaths seem beyond understanding. Some of the hardest grief work may be done in reconciling the ways loved ones have died. A spiritual view which recognizes that soul and spirit can already be out of the body before a violent death, and, therefore beyond pain, can be most consoling. Even in the most terrible circumstances of death, the soul and spirit can see heaven opening and angelic help reaching toward them as they cross over. The hard task of survivors may be to transform the images they may have experienced, and imbue them with spiritual understanding. Everyone is called upon to find greater insight, acceptance and forgiveness.

Regardless of the age of loved ones who die, they call for our recognition of their spiritual individualities that continue to be active and growing in another plane of existence.

C. S. Lewis, the famous writer and theologian, married late in life and was profoundly in love with his Helen. When she died from cancer, he was devastated. Yet with a deep, objective honesty, he watched his process afterward and wrote a remarkable book, A Grief Observed.* The writing is touching, penetrating, and hopeful, and written by a man who directly and deeply experienced the agonizing loss of a loved one. For him, as well as for many, such a death can be a critically defining aspect of our human experience.

C. S. Lewis describes how, after a period of intense grief, he arose one morning and found things had "lightened." The world seemed vivified with new forces. This statement makes sense, for when we are asleep, we have experiences in the spiritual world with loved ones who have died, and can feel sustained and inspired when we wake up.

He further writes,

> "for I have discovered, passionate grief does not link us with the dead, but cuts us off from them. This becomes clearer and clearer. When I feel my least sorrow, H. rushes upon my mind in her full reality, her otherness. Not as in my worst moments, all foreshortened and patheticized and solemnized by my miseries. But as she is in her own right...I will turn to her as much as possible in gladness...I will even salute her with a laugh. The less I mourn her, the nearer I seem to her."

He describes an experience with Helen one night as,

> "incredibly unemotional...the impression of her mind fac-

ing my own, not soulful...more like a practical phone call,...
intelligence and attention...extreme and cheerful intimacy,
yet so business like. Utterly reliable, firm. There is no nonsense
about the dead!"

*As we work through grief and loss of our loved ones, we are greatly aided by
the abiding knowledge that they are not truly dead. Rather, they have made a transition to a spiritual state of existence. A beautiful young woman I know described
her experience when her mother died in a plane crash. She was attending gradu-
ate school far away from the scene, and was enjoying a school picnic, surrounded
by a large group of friends, when the crash occurred. At the very moment her
mother died, a sudden flooding wave of light and love enveloped her. She felt overwhelming compassion and love flowing from her heart to her friends and the whole
world about her. She later knew, without question, it was her mother's presence,
loving her and, along with great universal love, preparing her for the news to come.*

*Too often we do not notice our connections across the threshold because they
can be very subtle, such as a gentle lifting of mood, a flood of gratitude, a perva-
sive joy at a beautiful concert, a sudden, crisp clarity of understanding, a child's
question, a joy-filled daily task, and all those times when we know the loved one
would have appreciated the moment. Above all, it is gratitude for the gift of that
loved one's presence in our lives, gratitude and love, and the remembrance of all
we loved and shared together that brings us closer to them. As C. S. Lewis writes,
"The presence of the beloved is ephemeral...charming...like someone laughing in
the other room." But the presence is there. As we work through our grief, we can
be ever more aware of the continuing connections between those living here and
those "living" on the other side.*

*Lewis, C. S., **A Grief Observed,** (N.Y. Bantam Books, 1976)

OUR CONNECTIONS TO THOSE WHO HAVE DIED

If we truly have a spiritual view of human development, then we count the threshold of death as a transition, not the final extermination of an individual. We can hold a faithful knowing of this truth, despite the anguish of separation we experience with a death. Awareness that the spirit continues, and is a presence in our lives, even though much less tangible than when the person was in physical existence, enables our thoughts and actions to follow accordingly. While the living presence of our loved ones on the other side can be subtle, it is an experience for anyone open to it. One of the most common experiences for those left here on earth is the appearance of the loved ones in dream, vision, or message telling them that they are "all right."

At death the soul and spirit are adapting to a new life without a physical body. Right after death, the one who has died experiences a life review, before moving on to a fuller experience of the life just lived. This process will take about one third of the time they lived on earth. We sleep about one third of our lives, and during sleep our life experiences go deeply into our spiritual organism. During this post-death time we bring up for conscious review the deeper impact of our deeds and life experience which we absorbed during sleep. This will be the time we measure what our intentions for our life have been, and what was fulfilled and what was not.

The experience of one who dies in old age will be different from someone who dies as a child. Children will stay close to the parents, giving their innocent presence as a bridge between earthly and spiritual life. They hope to work as inspirers, awakening the parents to the deeper spiritual aspects of life. The elders will always keep loved ones they have known on earth with them. They will follow their lives and development with interest. They can hope the ones left on earth can continue spiritual, cultural and social renewing impulses that they may have worked for in their lives. In spiritual existence, one can have an all-seeing awareness of life unfolding on earth, a broader and prophetic sense of the destinies of loved ones.

However, being un-embodied, there is no ability for the ones in spiritual existence to DO things. Only on earth can we do deeds, creative transformative acts that will effect change, and improve and give new substance into the unfolding life of humanity.

The impulses of the angels and those on the other side must flow through our acts, our hands, our deeds, our thoughts and our words. Together we can make incredible teams of co-workers; those with broad spirit vision on the other side, and we here on the planet where we can do deeds to effect a difference in the world. The world needs such potential working partnerships to become a conscious part of our lives.

The reality, however, is that there cannot be a flow of inspiration between those here and there unless it is on the wings of love, prayers, gratitude and continued remembrance of those who have passed on. Our thoughts of car repairs, shopping, making money on the stock market or cynical thinking that we are merely products of animals instincts and genes, are completely meaningless to those who have died. If we are constantly absorbed in materialism, there can hardly be a connection.

But when we daily turn our thoughts to spiritual striving and gratitude for life and all its beauty, through prayer, meditation, and especially through reading literature that embodies eternal spiritual truths, this becomes a wonderful sustaining nourishment for those on the other side. They are dependent on such conscious thoughts flowing to them from us. The reading need not be out loud, but it should be deliberate and thoughtful with our full attention. It is helpful if it can be given on a regular basis.

There are many other ways we can give them support. It is wonderful when we can recall them in detail, smiles, gestures, appearance, the way they walked, and so forth, and bring them close as we read, as we are experiencing a wonderful symphony, fine lectures, religious sacraments, works of art, nature in all its glory from sunsets to a perfect rose, butterflies and birds, weddings, festivals, and events of social communion. From all of these events we can share with them the uplifting of the soul that occurs at such moment. We find we can "pay attention" for them, as well as for ourselves.

There are times in our work when we are striving for the highest and best, when we feel everything flow, when ideas are there, when it is almost like another hand is guiding ours, or special words and thoughts spring to our mind. There we are "accompanied." One of the main ways our beloved ones on the other side communicate with us is by giving us thoughts, which we think are our own, which lead to new meetings, opportunities and awakenings.

Love knows no barriers. There is no threshold which can hold it back. We can be especially close to our loved ones when we recall those times when our hearts shared love, joy, laughter, and the appreciation of life and all that it means.

Gratitude is the most powerful soul force we need to remain close to those who have died. Gratitude for the gift of their acknowledgement and inspiration and the privilege of knowing them. With gratitude, we create a chalice in our heart, a warm and tender space where the love of our dear ones can make their presence known. With God we are never alone. When we strive to nurture our connection to those on the other side who have loved us, we can come to realize their loving care and concern is always present in our lives.

COMMUNITY THRESHOLD WORK

The stories in this section on community threshold work have been chosen to illustrate a variety of events that can occur around dying and home death care. This includes everything from inspiration about the importance of caregiving to difficulties with morticians and coroners, and some of the humorous aspects that can be part of the death care process. Two stories describe the spiritual grace that can be present even in deaths through violence and suicide. Another illustrates how our lower "double" personality can be transcended with the deed of dying and the last speaks of the life transforming changes that can come for family and friends through home vigils.

BEING THERE

At first this story doesn't seem to have anything to do with threshold work. But I am sharing it because in the end, for me, it had everything to do with it.

My husband Gordon is a pilot. At sixteen, before he had even bothered to get his driver's license, and with only four hours of instruction, he lifted a sleek little Interstate Cadet with feather light controls into the air alone. This solo flight began his life long love affair with flying, as it had for his father before him. It continues to this day.

After our marriage, he longed for me to share his passion for the skies. I was willing enough and, when opportunity came, I soloed a broad-winged, 65-horse, tail dragger Taylorcraft for my first thrill of flying independence. The dour, long-faced, gravelly voiced instructor, who turned me loose that day by simply walking away from the plane, had no idea I was pregnant. While I was keenly aware of the empty seat beside me as I lifted off, I was, in truth, more accompanied than I knew. Our twin daughters were born four months later.

After I was licensed, Gordon and I had friendly contests for the smoothest landings, and, one day at least, on a tiny, short and narrow tarmac airstrip with a tricky wind shear on the approach, I painted the landings on even more proficiently than he.

But Gordon also had another life long dream, to make a parachute jump. This was something I had certainly never considered myself. Then Lauren, our eldest college-aged daughter made a solo parachute jump. She did this with no preamble, and actually told us casually only after the fact. This was in the pre-tandem days when one came down alone and not strapped to an instructor guiding the descent. Her feat prompted a scramble of siblings to follow suit. Finally only Gordon and I, one twin, and the under-aged youngest son remained uninitiated in this thrilling new sport of skydiving. Somehow I really didn't want to miss out on sharing this challenging adventure with my husband and, with our 30th wedding anniversary on the horizon, our household of exuberant adolescents encouraged us that making a jump was just what we ought to do to celebrate. "Have a great falling out for the 30th!" they exclaimed, cheering us on. And so it was decided.

The anniversary morning dawned bright in May. We piled the family into the great box of a green Ford van and set out through sprawling California farmlands and down long country byways with names like Road 98 and Road 52 West. Finally arriving at a huddle of nondescript buildings beside an airstrip, we promptly began ground school.

The instructor spoke of wind speeds, reserve chutes, and techniques to control the jump. As we mounted a funky, four foot wooden platform to jump off for practice in thudding to the ground and then immediately rolling over, while curled in a banana-like position, my inner voice began to question the sanity of the whole enterprise. The great romantic notion of adventure, leaping into the skies with my beloved of three decades, gave way before sobering realities. At most, were we "taking undue risk with our lives?" At least, might I tweak a knee that could someday throb with arthritis on a daily basis to remind me of this wild escapade?

I was fifty-two years old. The chances of coming down, hitting the ground at great speed in clumsy combat boots and breaking an ankle seemed, well— excellent. Soon we were garbed in ill-fitting red and green coveralls. Then we waited and waited for calm winds which never came. Somewhat deflated (and I somewhat relieved), we drove home with a rain check for the following day. The kids chattered and bantered, but I rode in relative quiet, musing on the whole affair. Gordon's enthusiasm was not to be dampened, however. His brow was animated and his brown eyes alight with excitement as he looked forward to the event. Despite nagging questions to my better judgement, I kept silent. Morning came soon enough after a restless night. Mustering false and tepid enthusiasm, I downed breakfast with the crew and we were off again.

The spring day was crystal clear, beautiful in every way, and the winds were perfect. We suited up and in no time, lugging our gear, we piled into a high-winged six-place Cessna 205 with one door completely missing.

Jumping protocol requires that the heaviest jumper go first, which put Gordon, at 6'3' and 200-some pounds, in the jump seat, beside the pilot. Right by the missing door, he was cooled by the rushing slip stream, turned with his back to the control panel. The jump master squatted before him. Behind the pilot's seat was an open-faced young man sporting a crew cut who had never jumped before and somehow had been sandwiched in with our family for this event. I was crunched beside him while our daughter, Vivian, her fresh scrubbed, warm-eyed beauty aglow with eagerness, crouched across from us. Just then I envied her trim athletic youthfulness.

The excitement mounted as we climbed to 3,500 feet. It was time for Gordon to go. I could feel his anticipation. As he got his instructions, I caught his eye with what he told me later was "a small knowing half smile," and whispered, "I love you." I waved as he left the plane. The tension was incredible. As I crouched down on the floor of the plane, I couldn't see out the other side. I pleaded with Vivian to tell me if his chute had opened. It had. "Thank God," we sighed with relief. Whatever had possessed me to do such a jump and simultaneously worry about my family members!

It was now the young man's turn. He looked at me with vulnerable, candid eyes, full of fear and hope. He reached out and impulsively took my hand. In that moment I did not fathom the depth of all that lay behind his look. With bravado, I grasped his hand. "You'll do fine," I told him confidently as I was thinking, "Hey, you're young and strong, no problem." Out he went. It was my turn.

With the bulky chutes strapped on me, I scrambled forward to the hot seat by the door. The grey-haired jump master, warm and crisp but army-sergeant serious, gave me last minute instructions. Searching his face, I nodded. The pilot throttled the engine back in a slow turn above the drop zone where I saw a fifty-foot long, magenta-colored banner which the other kids had gleefully unfurled when we took off. Scrawled in three-foot high letters, their greetings were there for us as we came down, "HAPPY 30th MOM AND DAD!"

I swung out of the plane, my left foot on a tiny metal step, and both hands hanging firmly onto the strut, the brace that supports the wing. My right leg was swinging free in space, my body was buffeted and caressed by the ninety-mile-per-hour wind of the slip stream. There was no fear, only an exhilarated fascination with the kaleidoscope of fields rotating 3,500 feet below as we circled.

The moment ended abruptly with a nod and a command from the jump-master, "Go!" Every fiber of consciousness focused into my hands gripping the cool and solid metal of the strut, this fragile anchor in a sea of sky. The moment of truth had arrived, the threshold, the letting go, letting go of all safety, stability, the known, letting go and releasing into the unknown. My fingers opened, and I slipped away, falling back into the vast sea of space, the element of gracious air where gravity bound humans can but temporarily be at home. Will the chute work? In seconds the static line pulled the chute open with a firm jerk. The great canopy blossomed full and comforting above me.

Every sense was quickened to maximum levels as the world radiated below and around me. The spring green fields, the rich and textured hues, the warmed tans of brown plowed fields leaping vibrant to the eye, the airport small and beckoning, the air delicious, all were effused in a magical radiance of permeating morning sunlight. I looked up into the great white canopy as I hung suspended in this airy element of near weightlessness. Above, the chute seemed like a giant placenta nourishing and protecting my existence, mediating between me and the sun which poured its light through the canopy top. Filled with joy, I kicked my feet in exuberant freedom. Yes! This was as close as it gets, as close as it gets in these physical mortal bodies to the feeling of being free... free, like spirit! I now had the tiniest fleeting sense of how it must have been before we were born: like a drop of spirit held close to the sun in the womb of the cosmos. The crackling of the radio strapped at my waist broke in. A ground instructor asked if I was okay. "Yes!" He instructed me to move to the right and I pulled the toggle ropes, which rotated the chute. I was partly grateful for his attention and guidance and partly resentful at his intrusion into those fleeting moments of glorious freedom.

Too soon, too soon it would be over. The ground rushed up, fast. Inwardly mustering my knowledge of landing, I hit hard and rolled. I was down, and nothing was broken. Hallelujah! I reached to catch the chute before it could fill with wind and drag me, but the winds were calm. My daughter, Mary, her long brown hair flying came running and shouted, "Go, Mom!" as she traversed the plowed furrows of the field with graceful bounds and rushed to my side. She was at once solicitous and proud. Amidst joyful relief, my first question was, "Is Vivian okay?"

"Yes, she's coming down now." We both looked up into the sky to see a tiny form kicking happily away just as I had, under a huge white and orange canopy. Celebration! All up and all down safely. We hugged, cheered, chattered and compared. We teased about the finger prints left permanently in the strut of the plane where we had clung before letting go. Others gathered around to hear about this family saga and, of course, there were the triumphant photos.

But, as we gathered for the picture, the jumpmaster, George Morar, unbidden, came up and posed in the picture, too. He pushed right in, smiling confidently, as though he belonged there. Although slightly miffed that he was placing himself in our 30th anniversary family portrait, I could not bring myself to say anything. We congratulated all around and began the homeward trek, chattering all the way to the house for a gala party with friends. Now that fears for safety of life and limb were behind us, I began reviewing the experience with sober and objective detachment. Through all the hoopla, a part of me, like watching myself as a stranger, continued to re-play the event far into the night. Especially, I was drawn back to the moment just before I left the plane. More than once, as I crouched, back to the instru-ment panel, receiving the last words from the jumpmaster, I had made some distinct gestures, moving my head back and forth. Now I realized why. He had been wearing a helmet with a plastic visor over his face as he was going to make a jump at the end of the run as well. Because of the reflections on his plastic visor, I kept moving my head to try to see his eyes. Thus began the internal conversation.

"Why did I want to see his eyes?" I asked myself.

"Because the eyes are the mirror of the soul," I answered myself.

"Why did I want to see the soul in the eyes?"

"Because I wanted to see the spark of spirit light shining there."

"Why?"

"Because I could die in the next few moments, and this might be the last human being I would ever see in this life."

"So what were you trying to find in his eyes?"

"Affirmation. Affirmation of the spirit. Affirmation that the spirit is real, that the spirit lives, forever. No matter what." The revelation flooded my whole being. I was charged with knowing.

"So that's why I made this crazy jump!" I exulted. I realized then how the young man in his fear and vulnerability had turned to me for human touch and affirmation just before his jump. He needed someone to give him sup-port. I went through this experience, I was now sure, so I could bring home solidly, without a doubt, the knowledge that it greatly and humanly matters when someone is truly present for another person at the thresholds of life. If we only knew what it really means in the whole scheme of things! I was on fire to rush out and tell everyone, every friend and caregiver in the world, "Do you know how important you are?! Do you realize how much, on a deep soul level, it means to bear witness to the spirit by just being there for someone else in transition?"

I recalled my terror-filled awakening from anesthesia after a surgery, when I could hear everything but could see only blackness. I had pleaded for a nurse to come and pray with me. I remembered the blessed relief and comfort when she finally came. At the times of despair in a human life, when a friend is standing by, what a difference it makes. What an affirmation of our journey to have someone who is steady, caring, listening, holding, witnessing with human spiritual support at the thresholds-birth, baptism, graduations, divorce, job loss, illness, death. Every stage is a loss, a gain, and a transition to a new existence. Even when the one in transition cannot outwardly acknowledge the aid, this is surely one of the deepest human acts we offer to each other.

Filled with a flood of wonder for our common human ability to support and empower the higher humanity in another, I tried to share my new awareness of this abiding truth whenever I could with friends and family. Then, only a few months later, the accident occurred.

George Morar, our jump master, went up to do some skydiving with a group of friends. George was to jump first, but as he stood in the open door to go, his reserve chute, which was strapped to his chest, blew open and flew out the door. Why he did not follow the instructions he had so sternly given to all of us in ground school to go ahead and jump immediately if this occurs, we will never know. He was incredibly experienced with hundreds of hours of both jumping and instructing. But this fatal time, as his chute opened it became entangled in the tail section of the plane. The other men jumped quickly to safety, but the plane, with rudder and elevators jammed, was going down with George and the pilot. Too late to save his own life, but in time to save the plane and the pilot, he jumped out, freeing the chute from the tail, but without enough altitude for his main chute to open. And so he died, sacrificing his life for his fellow man.

I went to the funeral. What I learned there filled me with even deeper wonder about the whole affair. George Morar had a life-long love of flying and later sky diving. As a young soldier in World War II, under General MacArthur, he had been taken prisoner by the Japanese in the Philippines. Through long and horrible, inhuman months in the POW camp, he had been starved, overworked and degraded. As hundreds were dying around him, George tirelessly worked to keep up the men's spirits. It was George who sang the songs from home with all the verses, George who planned cere-monies and prayers around the deaths of comrades, George who clandes-tinely created celebrations to keep alive the memories of holidays—Thanksgiving, Christmas, Easter and the Fourth of July. He was a man for others who was able to live beyond his own despair to encourage and nur-ture, to care, and to act as witness for the spirit to his fellowman.

The true depth of the experience now dawned on me. Gordon's and my exciting and romantic adventure, which indeed remains a warm and hal-lowed memory and a treasured highlight in a long and striving marriage, now took on deeper soul meaning. In the broader scheme of things, George was not just a nameless and indifferent man whose eyes I had searched for that day. He was a deeply caring human being, and I have no doubt that it was also because he was who he was, strong in human spirit, that I was enabled to receive the revelation born of this experience.

With his dashing cavalier smile, George had connected himself to us, by "stepping into the family picture" scant months before the end of his life, thus creating a bond of destiny. We have carried his memory ever since. Through my threshold work, I have become someone on this side who knows that he is continuing his work on the other side, work that is just as impor-tant as keeping hope alive in the hearts of his fellow prisoners in a horrible war of long ago. In a destiny exchange for his profound gifts to me, I still send him thoughts of encouragement and gratitude, which will flow to him as long as I can remember and can share this story with others.

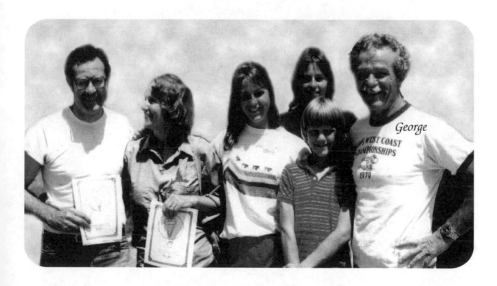

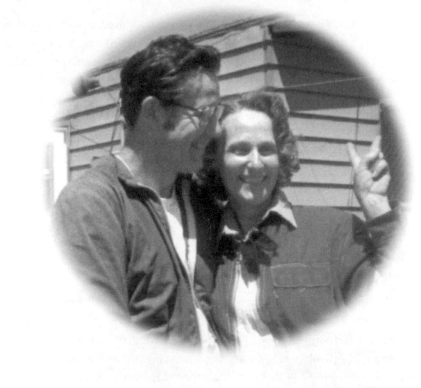

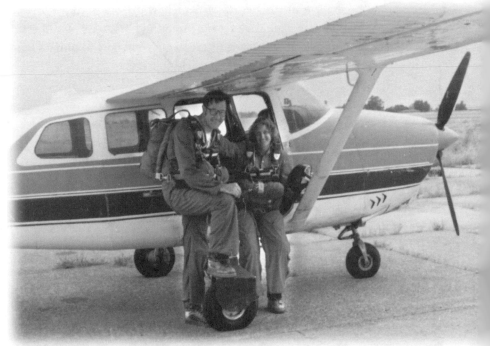

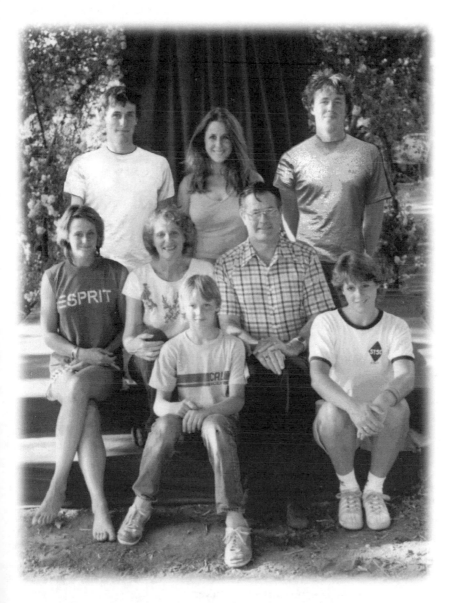

The family soon after the last grandparents transition.
Gary, Lauren, Cameron,
Mary, Nancy, Colin, Gordon, & Vivian

LENA

Joy and enthusiasm are the words I associate with Lena, but hers was a brief and challenging life. Her mother struggled for mental stability, and Lena, as a babe, was plagued with massive epileptic seizures and became retarded. She was put in a state hospital, confined to a crib, and heavily dosed with medication that never really controlled the seizures. She could not walk as her undeveloped legs were only able to hold her for a few seconds.

A state worker endeavored for over a year to place Lena in a small private care home where, in addition to providing physical care, the philosophy honored the spirit of each child regardless of his or her outer capacities. The effort was successful at last, and Lena arrived at the beautiful home to join five other children. She lived there for a few brief years that changed her life. In the end she could feed herself, play with toys, and make responses and eye contact with her caregivers—all major achievements.

The Easter of the year she died had been especially festive for the children. During the celebrations, with beautiful eggs, games, decorations and time outside in the lovely gardens, everyone noted that Lena was especially happy. She was unusually attentive and eager for the Easter stories and gospel readings. And she could walk! What a miracle that was! Though braced and wobbly and often needing extra support, her legs took her, by her own volition, where she wanted to go. Then four days after Easter, without warning, a massive seizure in the night took her across the threshold.

I awoke to the ringing phone late in the night and, in answering, heard a most poignant voice pleading for help. It was the nursing director of Lena's care home. She and another aide were at the mortuary. They had been pleading with the mortician not to embalm Lena's little twelve-year-old body which had already endured an autopsy. The autopsy was required by law because the death was unexpected. The man was harassing them unmercifully with his mortician's authority because they were making this request. The nurse was weeping. I could tell she was at the end of her rope and little wonder. Having already borne the shock of the death of a child in her care, she now had to face the scorn of an undertaker.

I got the man on the phone. He began his litany of why he needed to control where, how, and what happened with her body. I met him firmly and knowledgeably in his language. He finally lightened up. Inwardly I was furious with his attitude. Why, when caregivers are already shocked from a death, does such an attack come from an undertaker? Later the nurse told me that when he talked to me he "began to become a human being." But he should not have needed my confrontation. He should have been more humane and understanding from the beginning. The caregivers shouldn't have had to go through what they did.

Early the next morning I went to the home to pick up the child's clothes and heard the rest of the traumatic story. Lena had died in the night and, when they had called the authorities, a sheriff had arrived who treated the death as a possible homicide. This added even more hurt and shock to the experience for the distraught caregivers. Instead of being consoled, they were accused with questions. No wonder the undertaker was the last straw. I went to the mortuary. The undertaker didn't think the body should be viewed, but I insisted, and together we went into the back room.

Lena's slender body lay on the table with the great "V" of the autopsy whip-stitched in large brown sutures above her tiny breasts. She was just beginning to show the first budding roundness of puberty. Her eyes were blue, her lashes long and her soft fine brown hair swirled on the steel table. Her slender twisted hands and feet lay in stillness. She filled me with a tender loving remembrance of her valiant spirit.

The mortician began with excuses and explanations. I let him go on as I sought solutions to each problem he brought up. It was clear he was on the defensive and regarded his work as his province and scorned anyone who challenged his authority. If I could hold firm but find a compromise, things might work out. We discussed each aspect of the treatment of the body and the extent of the embalming. I left him with his authority intact, but the measures we wanted in place. We wanted to have the body back at the home for two days of closure and good-byes for all involved. She was to be dressed in the little overalls she had loved to wear.

It worked out. They brought her body back home. Now all who knew her could come and be in her presence and make adjustment to her new state of existence. Most importantly, all those around her could begin healing. They could honor and sing for the fair soul taken so suddenly from their midst. Community friends came day and night to pray and read scripture and poetry for the soul of the child, now freed from her hindered body and wide open to new experience in the spiritual world. The chapel for her service was filled.

Afterward, I looked back on her brief life and reflected on the incredible difference the few short years in the special home had made for Lena. She had been so tenderly cared for. All the children there were severely handicapped. Some could not even sit up. Yet in recognition of the spirit which existed beyond their handicapped bodies and minds, they were given "school." They were read stories full of depth and substance as though they could understand because it was felt on some level in their souls, they could understand. In addition to their physical therapy and care, they had songs sung for them, beautiful harp and flute music played for them, and food lovingly prepared for them.

They even had Sunday school. The service was given during the week because of all the time needed to bring them in to attend. I remembered a day not long before Lena died, when I was sitting in the back of the Christian Community Church, witnessing the service. The big transport van drove up bringing the six children with their wheelchairs and a kindly adult caregiver for each one. It was no small endeavor to organize all the lifts and transfers. On that sunny morning, I watched as the children were wheeled into their places before the altar. But that day Lena wanted to walk. She insisted on it. She was so excited and eager. She almost pulled away from the smiling, sturdy attendant who was helping her to balance her unstable steps. Lena was filled with determination to get down that aisle. She had such a joyful will and enthusiasm to be there and to make those wobbly legs do what she wanted!

The service was brief and gentle and filled with assurances of the love of God. Next to the church was a conventional daycare center. Inside the church were these severely mentally handicapped children with wobbly heads and ineffectual limbs. Yet one could feel every one of them straining inwardly with incredible concentration to take in the deepest meaning of the service. Meanwhile outside, the young day-care children screeched and yelled karate threats and curses to one another. I found myself musing which children were really "normal."

The kindly gray-haired priest was going down the line to shake the hand of every child. To each he would give the gentle solemn assurance, "The spirit of God will be with you when you seek Him." The child's response would normally have been, "I will seek Him."

Most of these children could not speak so each caregiver standing behind the child said the response, strongly and clearly for the child: "I will seek Him." Oh, how Lena struggled and uttered gutteral noises trying to make her own response! How radiant her face was as she returned down the aisle when it was over. How happy she was that day and through the days of the coming Easter time. She knew in the depths of her heart, "I will seek Him!" And, shortly after Easter, she did.

As my twelve-year-old son and I came back from reading for her after her death, he said, "She has a strong body now, and she will have one in the future."

"Yes," I replied.

"She's helped by all the 'praises,' " he said. Then he pondered, "Maybe that's not the right word?"

"Yes, son," I replied, " it's exactly the right word."

PICTURE STORY OF CHRISTIANA'S VIGIL

Our community threshold work included preparing a vigil for a beautiful baby girl, Christiana Marie, who died at home. Cameron worked through the night to create her casket. He told her family he felt she wanted it shaped like a crystal with a Celtic cross on top.

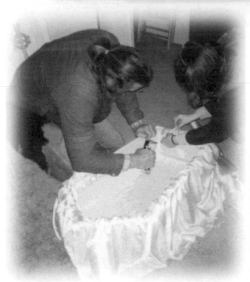

Preparing the pink silk cloth for the lining of the casket.

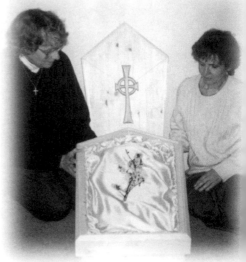

Christiana's godmother, Jannebeth, a nurse, helps me prepare the child and then her casket for the vigil in her family home.

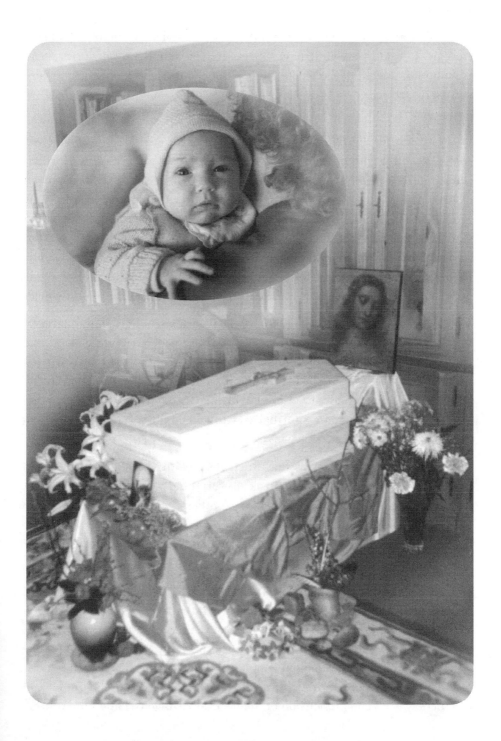

BELLE

Belle was from Texas. She had an expansive style, a combination of graciousness, pride and chutzpah. She didn't so much preside over social encounters, she simply reigned. With adroit charm she helped you realize you were privileged to be in her company—like royalty, or a proud native daughter of Texas.

Not that her life was privileged. She had hard scrabble times, widowed early on with young boys to raise, but none of it was too daunting for her. Bolstered by a penchant to see theater and humor in all things, she arrived at her needy years with courage, wry wit and royal tendencies intact. While a resident of a small nursing home, she would dress up in full makeup and elaborate hair styles for visits from her son and his gracious wife. Inspired by our care of Grandma Mary Edna for her death at home with the family, they wanted to do the same for Belle. Lorraine, Belle's daughter-in-law, made a special commitment to be with her for her transition across the threshold.

Once established at their home, Belle's care was alternately hilarious, fulfilling and maddening. For in addition to her considerable charm, she could also be insistent and difficult. After many months the family needed respite and Belle went briefly to a big nursing home and there, unexpectedly, died. Lorraine, who had vowed to be with her through to the end, was dismayed. But then she made a further vow to make Belle's send off everything it could possibly be.

The death occurred at a time when my health was flagging, so I told myself I would just stop by to check if everything was going all right, but would not really get involved. There were others who could help. So while running some errands with my eleven-year-old son, Colin, I stopped by where they were preparing for the vigil. It was in a picturesque garden house behind the doctor's office.

Belle's son was there. He was a pleasant, gray-haired counselor and teacher who had inherited her wit, charm, and restless sense of adventure. He and his wife greeted us warmly, both of them still in the open, vulnerable, sensitive wonder stage that can come with a loved one's passing. They had contracted with a cremation company to deliver the body from the nursing home. I began to inquire tactfully if the body had been prepared. I could see there was no comprehension of the necessities involved and I knew I certainly did not want to bring up the gross bodily needs to a man whose mother had just died.

Just as I was weighing the situation, two young men drove up with the body. They alighted and opened the back door of the van. Taking them aside, I discretely asked them if the body had been cared for at the nursing home. They didn't know what I was talking about. As they took the simple casket out, lifting it none too adroitly onto the ground, they tipped it sharply and there followed the distinctive and permeating odor of bowel fluid escaping. Exactly the problem I had been concerned about! Everyone stood frozen in a stunned silence. It became crystal clear I was going to be involved in this one.

So I tactfully dismissed Belle's son and the two fellows, who actually couldn't wait to leave, after we had them put the body up on a table in the garden house. "Well, here we go," I said and I went to look in the kitchen of the doctor's office for supplies. It was a weekend and no one was around and I could only find one rubber glove under the sink, along with some rags and Lysol (Normally we would pack the anus with cotton.) I was shaking my head with amusement. So much for trying to skip this one!

A nice lady came to "pay her respects" just at this awkward moment. There was nothing to do but explain the situation. Though this was all totally new for her, she seemed game for the experience, and Lorraine and I signed her up on the spot. Lorraine was overcome with the theater and drama of it all. It was so like Belle's inimitable style. "I knew she would do this to me!" she exclaimed.

So we went to work, getting the rags in place and some suitable clothes on Belle's body. Turning, wrestling, scrubbing, cleaning up—and laughing. There was simply no other appropriate response. It was Belle's last great joke and we might as well go along with it in good style. And we did. Three women at the threshold and Belle presiding from the spiritual world. It was a comical and remarkable time that sparks levity and laughter every time any one of us thinks about it, even years later.

My son who was with me had been blissfully shooting baskets in a hoop out in the yard all this time. When the body was ready to return to the casket we called him in. I asked him to take her feet for the lift, which he cheerfully did, and then went whistling outdoors again to shoot some more free throws.

So all's well that ends well. Belle's daughter-in-law was faithful to the end. Along with her husband, she attended Belle at the vigil with devotion and wonderful prayers, day and night, as did so many community friends. I returned at the end of the three days to a beautiful and sanctified space.

This vigil had begun with theatrics, tears, dismay and laughter, and the bald physical needs that come with death. Three days later, the expanding spiritual presence, created by Belle and all who had come to honor her, had filled the space with exalted peace and joy.* Lorraine was extraordinarily beautiful, translucent, transformed and radiant with spiritual light. In gracious reciprocity for her sacrificing gift of true service and caring, she had surely received the final truly royal blessings bestowed by her remarkable mother-in-law, the indomitable Belle.

*See **THREE DAYS AFTER DEATH—THE PROCESS**

OLD VICTORIA

Old Victoria was far older than she ever wanted to be. She had been try-ing to get off the planet for years. Not overtly, you understand. After all, she was Catholic and exhortation against suicide was laid solidly in her bones. But the harangue of wanting to die was constantly on her lips until almost everyone who heard her would roll their eyes and look the other way. Victoria couldn't wait to die, and she let the world know it.

Not only was it hard on her, but frankly, it was hard for many people to understand why she was still around. What for? Widowed and lonely, far from her native Italy, she lived in a modest home in the inner city and had a reputation in the neighborhood as the old harridan. Small and bent, gnarled and homely, she policed her front fence with a broom and epithets of scorn for the children who noisily and carelessly played there. In broken English she shrieked at them all and swatted those she was quick enough to reach with the broom. A friend of mine moved next door to her and, in a gesture of friendliness, brought her a bouquet of flowers. Not missing a crabby beat, Victoria immediately rejected them. She wasn't about to deviate a whit from the uniform negativity she displayed to the world, even for this unaccus-tomed gesture of kindness.*

But my friend was the persistent type and interested in threshold work. During a workshop retreat, she asked me what she could do for Victoria. I asked Victoria's religious background. "Catholic, from Italy," she answered.

"Well, you need to go where they are to give support," I told her. "The rosary would be familiar to her. Try to help her see that despite everything, she can still do the work for Mother Mary on earth. I believe some of these elders who seem to be leading useless lives are really helping society in spir-itual ways we are hardly aware of. As they near transition, they are no longer so tightly held by earthly goals and desires. They are already partly on the way to spiritual existence, and I feel many of them, especially those who can pray for others, can actually be holding the door open to the spirit for the rest of us who are too 'busy with life.' "

My friend reported that when she returned home it was no longer a dilemma for her. "I didn't actually say anything overtly to her," she told me, "but I was more at peace myself with it. My attitude changed. So I 'thought' things to her. I went and bought her a rosary in a second hand store. Something changed. She wasn't talking about dying all the time anymore."

As Victoria became more feeble, none of the neighbors wanted to help her except my friend. Victoria's reputation for meanness had built a solid moat around her, and nobody in close range was motivated to bridge it.

In the end she went to a nursing home, but it was a good one. She was well cared for. And there it all came around. The battle got fought—and won. Mean Old Victoria became sweet! Not only sweet but even adored by the nurses. They couldn't wait to be with her. She was beloved.

Somehow with the experience of being warmly cared for by others, Victoria was able to move through her own soul process. Her battle with her own double and lower nature that had so often claimed the upper hand was successful, and she came to master it.

When we see a helpless old invalid body, lying inactive in the bed, we cannot guess what soul battles are being fought inwardly. Never underestimate the dynamic situation in an old one! There is a drama taking place in the soul. It is working through all the life wounds, received, given, and self-inflicted: the bruising and lessons of life, the achievements, fulfillment and joys. All tumble together as the spirit threshes and winnows the destiny through to resolution and closure. It can be a wonder to witness the outcome.

Crabbed and cranky Victoria at last found her sweetness. The spirit won! Her treasure, lifted from the dross, was radiant and enchanting, and drew others close to warm in its light. Mighty stuff? You bet! This is great reward for staying the course, to find the victory in life—a process that can be sadly cut short when the option is euthanasia.**

Victoria died on Christmas Eve, the eve of the birth of the Holy Child she had always kept somewhere in her heart. My friend, busy with family herself for the holidays, intuitively got the call to go to her bedside. She went and stayed for two hours. Victoria's breathing was deep, peaceful and calm; then her eyes opened about a half an hour before she died.

"She looked at me," my friend related, "her blue green eyes all watery, and gave me a gaze I have never seen before. It was utterly indescribable. I then reassured her it was okay to go, that everything was fine, and she died."

"It is a glimpse into eternity," I told her softly. "You can see the same thing in the first hours of a newborn's life. The veil is lifted and, for a moment, it is as though you can spiritually see through their eyes into that incredible place of timeless existence, a place of eternal wisdom and love."

"Yes, that is it!" she replied excitedly.

I expressed my joy and thanks for the good threshold work and for her accompanying Victoria in her final hours.

"Yes, but I received so much," she responded.

"Of course," I replied, feeling gratitude for the deep and timeless goodness of their sharing. "She gave you the gift of experiencing her spirit at death, and you gave her your caring presence for the transition. A double blessing!"

"Even the young nursing aides who came to prepare her were filled with a reverence. They said, 'Remember she's still around us and can hear us,' " she told me.

Long ago, by the baptismal font of a Catholic church in an old village somewhere in Italy, a baby girl received her name, a name which means "to win in life." Nearly a century later, at the finish line, she fulfilled it. . . victorious Victoria.

*See **THE DOUBLE**

See **EUTHANASIA AND ASSISTED SUICIDE

KEVIN

Kevin lived swiftly and died young. As a child he was an intense, sensitive, boy with an easy compelling charm. He loved the outdoors, delighted in sailing and hiking, and was always game for adventure. But as the crucial years of early puberty years came, drugs claimed his life direction. By the reports of those who knew him well, he struggled to come to grips with the mundane demands of ordinary life and in the end remained on the borders of other realities that eventually led him into a life outside the law.

Like so many young people, Kevin had a deep longing for a world where everyone was accepted, where everyone had a right to be recognized and celebrated. That was how he lived his life socially. No one was outside his range of friendship; no color, race, religion, or class separated him from the people he wanted to know.

But trying to work with him was as erratic as trying to guess the next direction of a squirrel dashing across the road. When he was seventeen it became impossible for him to be at home. His mother never knew when she might see him. The last time she saw him, only a day or two before he died, he had seemed strong and powerful, even bathed in an extraordinary light. He told her he loved her. Two days later he was dead.

He died in a robbery attempt; by all accounts having gone further than he would truly have wanted to go: that is, actually to threaten the life of another human being. The victim fired in self defense and Kevin turned and ran, and then, mortally wounded, died in the arms of his friend and accomplice.

I received the phone call late on the night before New Year's eve. The distraught mother, stunned with the news, was desperate to have her son's body at home for the last time. She appealed for help.

So I began a series of phone calls to the coroner. Under the law, the next of kin has the right to disposal of the body. But it was a weekend and a holiday, and, with a minimal staff at the county office, no one wanted to deal with the case. Legally, they didn't have to supply the death certificate for three days. Yet it was just these first three days that meant so much to the mother and the community that wanted to support his transition with prayer, reading, and a vigil. I was persistent, hammering away through endless answering machines and delays, until I finally reached an authority on call for the weekend. Even though I was acting on behalf of his mother, I could not get them to release the body to her. I cited the law entitling her to this, and her religious beliefs as well. I was angry at their recalcitrance, especially since virtually anyone driving a funeral home truck could come up and get the body and take it away at any time.

They were probably dragging their feet for other reasons as well. Because it was a criminal case, an autopsy was performed with only prefatory repairs and minimal cleanup. They probably did not want the body to go back to a family without an undertaker's ministrations. Ultimately, we had to hire a mortuary to get the body, and it was released to them immediately, with no problems and no questions asked.

In the late afternoon of the first day of the New Year, I entered the back door of the mortuary, close by the crematory furnace, to find the body lying on a gurney. Kevin had been shot several times, and his hands, blackened with finger printing ink, were encased in plastic bags. The autopsy incision had been hastily closed. The skull was askew where they had taken brain samples. The repairs and cleanup would require strength and powerful solvents, more than I could manage at home.

While the undertaker and my son, Cameron, who had brought the casket, stood by, I slowly rolled Kevin's body over as I was making this assessment. But I was drawn to his face, which had not been injured. "He is so young, so very young," I thought. But his youth was not what ultimately spoke to me most powerfully. It was the expression on his face. A look of the greatest compassion was there, an almost Christ-like gentleness in the features, only enhanced by the crooked ridge of skull under thatches of brown hair-like a crown of thorns. A look of revelation, of "knowing at last" suffused the countenance. I felt in the presence of holiness. Overcome, I whispered inaudible thanks for the honor of this moment and marked it to tell his sorrowing mother. I sensed that while he would have many lessons ahead on his spiritual journey, that he also had experienced a tremendous revelation of awareness as he passed through the threshold of death. Death and resurrection.

On a practical level, I finished checking his condition and released the care of the body to the undertaker. After the mortician had done his work, Kevin's body was placed in a beautiful oak casket Cameron had made. Now the hair was neatly combed, the skull aligned and the hands well cleansed. All was in order for public viewing. But the tender fleeting expression was gone. It was now the face of a handsome young man in death.

I was grateful for the undertaker's talents that made it possible for Kevin's body to be at home. I worked quickly to arrange the room and casket in the living room in time for the droves of his shocked and grieving young friends to come to weep and pray, and to mourn and make closure, along with the family and others in the community. The church for the funeral was filled. The priest gave a warm, supportive and insightful eulogy of Kevin's brief inexorable journey of life.

We cannot always know the ways of an individual destiny. Some lives that seem beyond hope, may be endowed with soul progress and great learning that we cannot know. I only know in beholding the countenance of this young man, who could not live within the laws of society, that I was given a brief glimpse of laws of the spirit where the Great Giver of universal mercy and compassion can be present for us all at death.

THE HEALING POWER OF SPIRITUAL RITUAL

MARY AND HER COUSIN DAVID

They were a hard working, middle-America family from hereditary lines sprinkled with vivacious, capable women and men who took their parenting seriously. Like all families, they had their joys, sorrows and challenges. The parents were united in the devotion with which they raised their two sons, but became divided in their marriage. After thirty years of striving and struggling, it ended in a hard and painful divorce.

Their son David was a special favorite of his cousin Mary, who was seven years older. As a child, David was a beautiful boy with cherub cheeks and bright eyes, full of eagerness for life. He had always looked up to Mary, and as a young girl, she had felt she was his special caregiver and playmate. Though they had grown apart in adulthood, when he decided to marry, David had called her to let the companion of his childhood be the first to know.

David was bright, warm, sensitive, impulsive and ambitious. He set his sights on achieving it all and he did: college, career, financial success, marriage, and a child. Then there were long bouts with alcohol, months in rehab, a second marriage, and in the end a fortune, millions made in the computer world as he applied his brilliance to cyberspace. Yet despite this outer success, no one could know the pain or circumstances surrounding his next step. At thirty-three he took his life.

Mary called me when the tragedy occurred.* She told me that in her last conversation with David, he had shared his happy memories of the years they had been playmates and friends, and she was deeply touched. Then we talked through the practical and spiritual aspects of the situation now. She weighed whether to leave her two young children to go back for the funeral many miles away. It had been twenty-five years since she had left her large, Midwestern clan, and she had been a child at the time. She wondered if her presence there would make a difference.

As an adult, Mary and her mother, David's aunt, had shared a mutual path of spiritual work which included reading and praying for those who have died. When David's father heard of this, it struck a chord. Mary's suggested that the extended family be called to read for David. All across the country grief stricken family members went to their Bibles and found quiet times to read the Gospel of St. John for David, whose very name means

83

"beloved." With this the family's sorrow was given direction and a sense that, together, they might offer him support.

Mary decided to go to the funeral. She arrived expecting only to aid quietly in consoling family members. However, awareness of her wisdom to help in this family crisis had preceded her. As she entered the room to join the family she had scarcely seen for so many years, David's father asked her to lead them all in a prayer circle.

Mary was taken back, a little shocked and surprised. While she was a capable kindergarten teacher in one of the international Waldorf schools, she was reserved in nature and had never taken such a ritual responsibility with adults. Yet out of deference for these elders, who were in such obviously bewildered pain, she felt she had to do it. In fact, everything she needed was at hand for a friend had put her on the plane with a Bible and candles in her suitcase.

Taking a deep breath, Mary reverently lit the candle and opened the Bible. After a beginning reading, she passed the Bible around so each one could add a voice to the circle, a circle bonded through pain and grief, regret and anger, and the shame and helplessness that such deaths leave in their wake. Now together they could do something. Each brought forth his or her voice in the timeless words of consolation, *"I am the light of the world; he who follows me will not walk in darkness,...Father, the love with which thou hast loved me may be in them, and I in them...to all who received him, who believed on his name, to them he gave power to become children of God...For God so loved the world."* Hope leavened the pain.

The next morning, when David's mother, Elaine, awakened for her son's funeral day, she prayed above all for a "circle of love." She knew the potential tension that might arise with David's father when they would meet at the church service. Yet on that day they bravely transcended their differences. They were able to sit together, to hold one another and to aid each other to the podium to speak to those assembled for the service. The father spoke a few broken, sorrowful words, thanking everyone for coming, Elaine, bare to the heart, spoke out, "David was a child of God. He wanted to live. He was overcome."

After the funeral, Elaine approached Mary and said she had heard about the prayer circle and wished she had been there. As the guests departed, and a smaller group gathered to comfort her, Elaine turned and asked Mary to lead them for a prayer circle. This time Mary did not hesitate. As she lit the candle, she was unexpectedly inspired to sing the song she sang for her kindergarten children each day.

"I can light a candle, God can light a star,
both of them are helpful, shining where they are."

As Mary's gentle, soulful voice sounded the notes into the room, Elaine cried, "Oh, that is beautiful, please sing it again." And so she did. Then Elaine asked, "What do you do next with the children?"

"I tell a fairy tale", Mary replied.

"Then tell us," the group urged her. What an amazing turn of events! Mary had never anticipated her kindergarten work would find a place here. There was nothing to do but go with the unfolding requests. She had recently memorized the story of *The Frog Prince* or *Iron Henry* for her kindergarten class. She took a deep breath and began.

"In olden times, when wishing still helped, there lived a king whose daughters were all beautiful but the youngest was so beautiful that the sun itself, which had seen so many things, was always filled with amazement each time it cast its rays upon her face."

As her words flowed softly into the space, Mary looked at the circle around her. The elders' life-worn faces, now sadly etched with the new pain of David's passing, were open and vulnerable. They were receptive and heart ready, their souls in their eyes, and scarcely different from the open wonder of the innocent children for whom she usually told the timeless story.

The magic of the healing imaginations in the fairy tale began to cast its spell. Mary's voice, at first tentative, became quiet and steady, as she unfolded the story of the princess and her love of her golden ball which had fallen into the deepest well where a frog with a thick, ugly head promised to return it if she would become his companion. Mary then told of the careless desertion of the frog by the princess and of how the frog knocked at the palace door to insist on being with the princess. When the princess tried to reject the frog, the stern warning came from her father, the king.

"If you've made a promise, you must keep it. Go and let him in."

Mary continued in slow, rhythmic tones as the vivid pictures of the eternal struggle for the transformation of the human soul unfolded.

"and the princess threw the frog against the wall with all her might. However, when he fell to the ground, he was no longer a frog but a prince with kind and beautiful eyes."

No one could have rescued the prince from the well and broken the spell save the princess, and

"in the next morning, when the sun woke them, a coach drawn with eight white horses came driving up. At the back stood Faithful Henry, the young king's servant. He had been so distressed when he had learned his master had been turned into a frog by the spell of the wicked witch that he ordered three iron bands to be wrapped around his heart to keep it from bursting from grief and sadness."

The tale ended, describing how the prince was alarmed as they drove away when he heard, three times, a great cracking noise behind him where his faithful servant stood on the coach,

"but the noise was only the sound of the three bands snapping from Faithful Henry's heart, for he knew his master was safe and happy."

The room was very quiet. Mary then brought it to a close, leading the group in crossing their arms over their hearts in a gesture of reverence, and recited the kindergarten closing verse:

"From my head to my feet,
I am the image of God
From my heart to my hands,
God's own breath do I feel.
When I speak with my mouth,
I shall follow God's will.
When I see and know God,
In my father and mother
In all loving people,
Then no fear shall I feel,
Only love that can fill me
For all that is around me.

The silent, healing moments that followed were profound. Mary's gentle words, united with the love of everyone there, and surely the spiritual presence of David, had woven a sacred mantle over them all.

After dinner the next evening, a smaller group of the usually lively and fun-loving family, now subdued with pain, adjourned to the patio of the hotel where most of them were staying. Friends and relatives joined them. It was time for good-byes.

Among the group was a girl of fifteen, also a cousin of David's. To Elaine and Mary, she quietly confided that she, too, had thought of suicide.

"I didn't do well my first year in high school," she explained, "so how can I do well and finish high school? Then I couldn't go to college, and couldn't make a lot of money, so what would be the use of being here at all?"

Her words stung. The young girl was mirroring the heartless, market-driven view of human worth held up by the media culture on every side. Like a slender reed braving a storm of materialism, she confessed her struggle to know her own uniqueness and find a purpose for living.

Shaken anew, Elaine grasped the girl's and Mary's hands to form a circle and said urgently, "We must pray about this now!" Embraced by two loving relatives, the girl found the words, haltingly, hopefully, "Please give the family strength, let us be together. . .help me not to give up." Her voice got stronger at the end. They joined the waiting family.

Then suddenly someone suggested they all sing, and sing they did. Pent up emotions flowed into their songs, urgent with warmth, and good, strong voices that echoed the happier times of a family that loved to dance and be together. At Elaine's special urging, the young girl sang a solo, and her pure, sweet voice seemed angel-like as it floated over the group. They cheered, urged her to sing more, and wrapped her in hugs of warm appreciation. In closing, Mary lit the candle for the third and last time and they ended with voices blended into rich harmony *"Abide with Us, Oh, Lord, and bless our new beginning of wisdom, harmony, health and joy."* For countless American families in such times of crisis, many turn to alcohol for support. But in these special three days it was spiritual solace that sustained them.

When Mary returned home and shared the story with me, she thanked me for "being there with her through it all," and told me, "Nancy, it was bigger than me, far beyond what I am." I smiled and replied, "Mary, it is an amazing story. Remember and hold it. You have experienced directly the deep well in the human soul that yearns for the spirit. Your gift has been given like a balm needed by longing souls of all ages everywhere. You've been able to see the power of sacred ritual that can fill that vulnerable space with true spiritual substance. It is truly a sharing in the work of the holy spirit."

It is a beautiful thing to watch someone come of age in her own extended family circle. I know that Mary daily pledges herself to her work with children with a prayer "to be a helper of humanity, a servant of sacred things, selfless and true." Like Faithful Henry to her cousin's painful transformation, she became his emissary, aiding him to do all that he might do in spirit to inspire the "circle of love," his mother longed for, between the spiritual world and life on earth. Mary had thought she would attend this event only to give quiet support for family. Instead she was central to a sacred healing circle, and her gifts, the fruit of her spiritual path, helped lift many there in three grace-filled days of spiritual community. She did indeed fulfill her prayer to be *"a helper of humanity, a servant of sacred things, selfless and true."*

*See **SUICIDE**

INITIATION BY SUSAN

A good friend died swiftly and unexpectedly, and she certainly was not all that old. The cancer moved with a remarkable speed that left everyone stunned and unprepared. But my dying friend met it head on. A powerful and tender woman, she had given a lifetime of care to others through her profession as a psychotherapist. After the doctors told her, she never went near the hospital. Surrounded by concerned family and friends doing all they could for her comfort, she stayed home, ordered a family picture and her own casket, and had a garage sale. It was only two weeks from diagnosis until she died. "Susan," I said admiringly as we spoke of her impending transition, "You are a cosmic event!"

I flew down to her home at her death to help create the vigil and life celebration as she had requested. I prepared the space in her bedroom, made it beautiful and practical for people to come, cared for the body, arranged it in the casket, and worked with the family. In preparing the body, I usually do not apply cosmetics unless there are unsightly blemishes. The state of death is natural in itself and it is not a state of life. But I realized in Susan's case that she had always been particular about her appearance and did not go out in public without makeup or her hair professionally done. Though her hair was now combed and neat, it was not the way she usually wore it. I also realized that these cosmetic factors were particularly hard for her young adult children who were painfully struggling to deal with her sudden transition. I knew I would need to make some changes.

There is almost always an auspicious timing of occurrences in the days right after a death. So often just the person or the thing that is needed appears, as if magically conjured up by the wish. This time was no exception. Just as I assessed the need and felt my lack of skill to meet it, Susan's hairdresser came to the house and knocked on the door. She was a young attractive woman in her forties, with pale brown hair and small capable hands. She was already stunned to find out that Susan had died so suddenly, and now she was further shocked to find the body was actually there in the house. It was clear she was more than a little frightened to see it as she had never had an experience with death.

I welcomed her warmly with expressions of hope that she would choose to help us. I told her she had come just at the moment she was needed. I explained that all was proceeding according to Susan's wishes, with a home vigil, prayers and a service with family and friends attending. I told her about how the individual who has died can be experiencing the transition in these three days. She was fascinated, breathless and attentive. At the same time, she was tremulous with the possibility of actually facing death. A friend, who observed the exchange, later told me at this point I audaciously said to her with cheerful tones, "Oh, then it is time to grow up!" I told her I would take her to the edge of the room and she could freely make a choice as to what was right for her with regard to viewing the body. I assured her that whatever her decision, it had to be right for her. We came to the door of the room with reverence. Another woman was standing quietly beside the casket. I left her there at the threshold.

She went over to the casket. Not only did she touch the body, but seeing the state of the hairdo, within minutes was fixing it and applying makeup. Within minutes! Ten minutes later, with her deceased friend's hair and countenance made more beautiful by her touch, she came out. She was a changed woman. She couldn't stop talking. She was amazed. She was fascinated. She was full of questions. Within an hour's time she had gone from wondering why on earth anyone would do anything so bizarre as having a body at home, to wondering why everyone didn't do it! The powerful strength that came into her in this brief time, in what was certainly a major life experience, was exciting to witness. One felt Susan had surrounded her with the nurturing love and energy of a cosmic midwife, birthing an initiation to a new state of awareness. Without doubt, I knew I was witnessing a palpable new confidence in her that hadn't been there before.

She left much later, after a very long conversation. She had come to the door of Susan's home, saddened and tense with trepidation. She left enlivened and stronger, having experienced the priceless gift given by Susan with her death, a gift so beautifully acknowledged by a client who said, "Susan opened doors for me I didn't know could be opened and gave me the wings to fly through."

Susan with husband Bob and daughter Rose

See **THE THREE DAYS AFTER DEATH—THE PROCESS**

A SPIRITUAL VIEW OF DYING
II

COMA

It is a common perception that people in a coma are completely unknowing and cannot be aware of what is done around them. Yet this view only considers the physical aspect of the human being. The soul and spirit are also involved and can be present in varying levels of awareness, from a state of preoccupation to a supra-consciousness, especially near the moments of death.

Spiritually seen, during a coma the soul and spirit are largely expanded outside the body and can be present with heightened sensitivity and receptivity. Most people can recall how it feels to be very ill and how sensitive their organism is in that state. Loud noises and sudden harsh moves by those around them can be felt like a shock. When someone is ill or dying, sharp and angry statements and abrupt physical movements can be experienced painfully, for such gestures can penetrate us more deeply in our expanded vulnerability than when we are all contained within our skin, so to speak. One can only feel great sadness for the awful events that sometimes take place around the death bed when families quarrel and jealousies and arguments ensue over money and possessions. The pall of bitterness is bad enough for the living, but tragic for the dying person who can be aware of the conflict but helpless to respond or to reconcile the problems.

When caring for bedridden and dying patients, we naturally have to meet their physical needs. We have to deal with cleanup, changing sheets and catheters, getting them fed, and so forth, all of which involves care and conversation. But if we are able to keep an awareness that the person is present on some level, even if outwardly it is not apparent, then we can truly serve in the most respectful and helpful way. Of course, it is perfectly normal to become exhausted and to want to say, "Oh, no, another mess just after I got the first one cleaned up!" but we can try to bring to the moment as much objective, matter-of-fact cheerfulness as we can. It is our good will to care for the patients that is perceived through their increased capacity to measure our soul mood as we render the care.

When considering the possibility of heightened awareness in a person in a coma, stories of near-death experiences would certainly seem to give extensive substantiation of the phenomena. The super-sensible perceptions experienced when people have nearly died and are then revived have now been described by over ten million people throughout the world. These are individuals of all ages, and from different ethnic and religious backgrounds. In these situations, not only is the person in a coma, but he or she is often not even registering the basic vital signs of life. Yet these people can, when revived, accurately report what was going on around them while they were physically inert. They can factually describe who was in the room, the procedures used to revive them, what time it was, what was said, and so on. Consciousness transcends the physical condition of the coma or near-death condition, although most people don't remember much later on. The eternal spirit of the individual knows and is supported, or not, by the consciousness of those around them.

A priest related the following experience to me. He told of coming daily to the bedside of a young woman who was in a coma for six months and reading the Gospels to her. When she recovered, she thanked him and told him what an incredible support these timeless words had been for her throughout her ordeal. The priest told me further of a young soldier during WW II who was critically wounded and taken to the hospital in a coma. Far down the hall from his room, a young nurse expressed sympathy for him, saying she did not feel he would live through the night. Super-sensibly, the young soldier heard her words, and the statement galvanized his will to live. "I will make it!" he vowed. He did recover and was able to recall the circumstances.

Think of what such experiences can mean to us. It means we can send love and prayers even from afar to loved ones and to those who are ill. What a comfort also when one arrives at a time just before death and the individual has already gone into a coma. So many people report despite the coma, "I knew she knew I was there," or "I could tell he heard my voice," or, "It was like she was waiting for me to come." All true.

Our thoughts can reach through to support our loved one who is in a coma, especially at death because of the dying one's expanded awareness. The thoughts and words do not need to be verbally spoken, though they can be, of course. Prayers, expressions of love, gentle singing, and gestures of forgiveness can be silently exchanged. Do not worry if there does not seem to be an outward response. Such caring is never in vain. Though it can seem somewhat strange to sit beside a quiet and seemingly sleeping person and communicate, it is not only possible but can be a priceless opportunity to give love, support and reconciliation at the time of death when we might have thought we no longer had a chance to do so.

THE DOUBLE

Anyone with even elementary self-knowledge, can recognize we all have a higher and a lower self. When we act from our higher self, there is a sense of clarity, generosity, warmth, love and goodwill. When we act from our lower self, we feel driven, instinctual, selfish, manipulative and harsh.

This lower or "double" aspect of our make-up, is no respecter of freedom, our own or anyone else's. Our double wishes to dominate others, but as we are dominating, we are certainly not free, for we are being compelled by this lower nature. Therefore, we can hardly come from a place of objectivity and a sense of bringing the higher good to the situation. On the other hand, one could say that all the stuff of the double and the lower nature is primal substance for conscious transformation by the higher self. Certain aspects of the double may be even a spiritually chosen challenge. While the lower double nature is very complex and uniquely personal for each one of us, there is also a generic aspect to it that all human beings share.

In order to be here on earth, we need an aspect of our nature that compels us into physical material existence. We need a strong pull to come from a body-free spiritual existence into gravity and earthiness. The double acts like ballast in a ship to keep us grounded and focused here. It binds us to matter. It stands behind our intellectualism and materialism, our capacities for dealing with worldly issues. In short, it is a necessary part of our make-up. There is, however, no redeeming conscience or warmth displayed where the double is involved. When this aspect of the individual dominates, one can experience a person who is cold, calculating, harsh and destructive. Carl Jung speaks of the "shadow" side of the human being though in a somewhat different context. Elizabeth Kubler-Ross often refers to our inner Hitler and inner Gandhi, aspects of the lower and higher selves. The native Americans tell us, "You have a twin brother whom you have wondered about and whom you would seek,...This I tell you: he is your other side in all things and in all ways. He is with you...do not seek him. Do not wish to know him...but <u>understand</u> him."*

Throughout history and literature, many examples are given of individuals who were unable to master their doubles and brought destructive forces into the world. However, in this brief essay, we are only considering the double with regard to dying.

95

As we age, we may have less mastery of our personality as the spirit begins to loosen its grip on the organism. It has less mastery of the bodily instrument. Unless we have made a deeper commitment to acting out of moral goodness, and have carried out a life of spiritual striving or religious dedication, the double can surface. Sometimes, even if we have worked for the good, we may become difficult and recalcitrant as the lower self acts out. We also have a lifetime of attitudes and habits we have built up, and the destructive side of these can be more exposed as we age. Working with elders and the dying can be extremely difficult when their doubles are lashing out. It is not their true being. Their behavior is often aggravated by brain damage, pain and depression, the loss of their loved ones, frustration and the loss of physical independence. We need tremendous objectivity to keep our equilibrium in some of these cases and realize it is their problem. They need clarity, common sense and empathy from us, not a fight. It is a profound social deed when we can faithfully hold a memory, an image of what we know to be their higher selves, during these difficult episodes.

Realizing how the dynamic of our behavior can manifest in either higher or lower aspects of our nature is a tremendous motivation to work on ourselves spiritually, from a young age on. I often say, "Whatever you are, when you are older, you are going to be more of it!" It is a worthy goal to strive to become an elder who can bring peace, wisdom and blessing to others.

Death is an act of the human spirit. It is an act of breaking free of the double, free of matter as the individual directs his or her own birth into another dimension. As we die, the earth-binding forces that keep us tied to our body cannot dominate the process. They have to give way before it. This can happen in a noticeable shift immediately before death, or up to three days before death occurs. Sometimes a general transformation can also be experienced in the last weeks before the transition. The weakening body can become more transparent and the spirit can shine through. Though the body can be nearly wasted away, it is often possible to experience a luminescent, transcendent quality of the individual, beyond mortality.

In some cases, the struggle to overcome the double is a severe one. We are not, after all, just old vegetables that merely fall off the vine. There is individual spirit intention as the dying one is striving to break free into spiritual existence. There is an active will seeking the chosen death moment. Rudolf Steiner states that if we could only see this moment from the spiritual side, instead of the often agonizing specter of the human physical side being played out, it would be an experience of the greatest inspiration. At death, the spirit comes forth like a magnificent flame, filled with power, light, and beauty. No longer confined to a physical organism, its brilliance provides a continuously guiding light to the individual in his or her new existence. It remains a wondrous reminder that the spirit has been victorious over physical matter.

In a case of intense struggle by the dying one to get free of the body, a struggle which can include the fear of dying, those attending the death can give aid with prayer, soft touch (when it is wanted), singing, gentle live music—such as a lyre, candle light, a communion service or other sacraments and last rites, and an atmosphere of positive encouragement. One has to be intuitive about just what can be the most supportive for the dying one at any given time in the process. They are engaged in the hard work of dying. They need space, quiet, and respect for their task. Being nearby with calm, attentive, prayerful support is always helpful at any part of the dying process.

The signs of becoming free of the double just before death can vary. In hospice work this phase is called appropriately "lightening." However, many caregivers do not recognize that these signs can also spell imminent death. When a person is in a coma, the signs will be more subtle, but those close to the dying one can often sense a deeper peacefulness, and more of a natural flow with the breathing and moving on when the double is gone. In other cases, there can be dramatic changes. An individual who has been mortally ill will suddenly seem to recover. He or she may have new strength, even appetite. Individuals who have been paralyzed with a crippling illness will often move and sit up, and sometimes even stand. I'm told my great-grandfather, lying sick abed, got up, pulled on his boots and went out and died in the barn. Dr. Naomi Remen, in her book, Kitchen Table Wisdom, *tells of a remarkable death in which the man had Alzheimer's. In fact, the autopsy following his death revealed his brain had been nearly destroyed by the disease. He had been unable to speak and communicate for nearly ten years. But, as he fell suddenly to the floor, with a fatal heart attack, he spoke out clearly to his son who was beside him. "Don't call 911. Tell your mother I love her. Tell her that I am all* right." Other such patients, unable to communicate for years, have, in the last moments, suddenly spoken clearly to loved ones, thanking them for all their care.

When the double is gone, the dying person may talk of going home, of taking a trip, of making new plans or of moving to another place. In reality they have been relieved of earthly burdens and the true spirit is now striving to speak. A state of elementary innocence and newness may be restored. Their voice can have a quality of child-like wonder and expectation, for they are already living into the future.

This is why death bed pleas for mercy, religious conversion or forgiveness need to be seriously honored. Now the true self, unencumbered by the lower self, even with someone who has dealt harshly with others in life, is trying to come through. We may be more open to the spirit in this moment than any other time in life. This is also why the privilege of being in the presence of the dying can be so great. We can stand before the spirit when it is the most radiant and real.

From the Mishomis Book "The Voice of the Ojibway," by Edward Benton Bansi

EUTHANASIA, ASSISTED SUICIDE, SUICIDE

Today there is a large group of people whose influence touches many, espe-cially educated individuals, who claim suicide and euthanasia are appropriate choices for "the good death." Appealing to individuals' desire to "be in control," and to their desire for comfort, for avoidance of disease, aging, and pain, and for limiting financial costs to the estate, such arguments are made to sound so very sensible. In a world view of pure physical materialism, they would seem rational.

But the spiritual reality is a far different story. Spiritually seen, we should ask, "What is gained from illness or dying?" Our inner intentions for our life can lie far deeper than our outer expression of desires to be comfortable and unchallenged. Elizabeth Kubler-Ross, who stands as one of the most experienced and insightful individuals who has worked with the dying, states she never had someone who was cared for that really wanted to commit suicide. She stands adamantly for loving care, not the elimination of the person. Needless to say, Mother Teresa took the same view.

Understanding that we take our soul and spirit with us through death gives a whole different orientation to the process of dying. Can we consider how someone working through an illness can also be going through tremendous soul transfor-mation? A purging of desires is in process. Reorientation of values, a cleansing of addictions and hatreds, and opening to new and universal understanding are all possible. When we go down a city street and see signs that say "Men at Work," we can expect to see active, hard hatted crews paving, shoveling, bulldozing, etc. in vigorous activity. If we could put up a sign at the sick bed that said "Human Spirit at Work," maybe we could develop more respect for the activity of working it through on a soul level.

How different is death when we have worked through things before we die, releasing, transforming, preparing, making closure and peace, forgiving, and shed-ding the desire-filled body for a new state of existence. Surely our angels will not give us more than we can truly bear.

We can ponder the wisdom of remaining in earthly existence when we see an incapacitated elder hanging on and on and ask, "Why?" (Here I am not speaking of aggressive life support interference at the end of a long life.) But if we can imag-

ine a spiritual picture of the catharsis that can take place through an illness, bringing the individual to a new state of consciousness and readiness for a spiritual existence, we come to a different view. It must certainly be recognized that the care givers are an integral part of the process, for they can be receiving deep human gifts for their own development from the dying one who is moving through the different levels of resolution.

It is my perspective that some elders are really holding a spiritual balance in the world today. With so many people locked into the grip of materialism and under the tyranny of intense desires and addictions, those who have lived beyond these obsessions can act as conveyers of spiritual goodness into the life stream of humanity. In the same way an infant at birth opens the door of the spiritual world and allows a flood of love and innocence to flow into our social existence, so too, an elder can help hold open the door on the other end of life, letting peace and perspective flow through, despite the struggles of existence, as a gift for all.

Suicide

One of the most poignant and difficult issues in human life is suicide. The reverberating pain that can echo from this deed is one of the most monumental sufferings in human existence. This can be the experience of those who are left, as well as for the one who has died. We can have empathy with someone facing a seemingly impossible situation. No one in good conscience can advocate impossible suffering. But the ending of life through euthanasia or suicide is clouded with problems.

The whole realm of suicide is a gray area. What is a true suicide? Often we don't know the inner soul condition of the one who has died. Was the individual "out of him or herself"? Was the person "beside him or herself'?" The very language tells us that the spirit, the higher self, may not have been in command of their actions. Certainly disorientation through drugs and alcohol is a common component in suicides. We can understand someone driven to despair through depression, pain, or blindly following others (i.e., epidemics of adolescent suicide). Therefore, we can aid those who have died in this way by holding them with the most positive thoughts possible, including the benefit of a doubt regarding their decisions.

The tragedy of suicide is the belief that it will end all the problems and pain. This is the materialistic view, that we cease to exist, we "get out." But this is far from the spiritual reality. You can kill the body, but you can't kill the soul and spirit. That is just the point! Soul and spirit go on. But how? The soul that continues beyond death still holds all the untransformed passions, addictions, sufferings, instincts, urges, hopes, ideals and desires that it had in earthly life. With the elimination of the body, there is no possible way to satisfy those urges and passions, or to transform them. The soul is tormented with desires that cannot be fulfilled, for there is no body to fulfill them. A "purification" is needed. This is spoken of in all religious traditions. The experience of the soul through this intense process will take time.

Interestingly enough, the one who commits suicide is often more attached to the body than others, and wanting more from life than they feel they are receiving. They are often caught up inside the walls of their own negative perceptions of life. The threat to the physical body of disease, pain or age (such as in the case of Ernest Hemingway) can hardly be tolerated. Yet in taking their life, they find they have eliminated a part of their being to which they were actually deeply attached and then must make an enormous adjustment on the other side. For this reason, it may be helpful if the body of a person who has committed suicide not be cremated. In a natural death, the body has been preparing for the separation of body, soul and spirit. With suicide, this preparation has not taken place. The person is suddenly thrown into another existence. It helps to have the body remain longer as a point of reference on the earthly plane as the individual adjusts to a new existence.

The person committing suicide has rejected the gift of life and entered the spiritual realm prematurely, out of season. The desolation of being in a limbo for a time can be one of great loneliness. In reports of near-death experiences, often those who attempted suicide and returned to life have not had the uplifting, light-filled meetings that are reported by the majority of those with near-death experiences. Some have reported great darkness and lower beings, and most will never try it again. It is a view held by many who hold reincarnation as a world view that only once in all lifetimes might an individual seek this type of death. Many who have tried suicide out of despair and been brought back to life can, through this threshold experience, find new resolves and a deeper meaning for living.

Everyone has known someone who has made a choice for suicide. In modern life, it can seem at times that it is not worth going on living. But we have opportunities for transformation here on earth as in no place else in the universe. So the situation of suicide calls for the greatest love, compassion and forgiveness that we can summon. Life will go on here and beyond. It is good to hold that person as objectively and clearly as possible so the restless soul of the suicide does not impact our lives unduly. We need to give unconditional warmth and support to ourselves as well as those who have died by suicide. We could not alter their choices and need to release them to their journey of learning. The raising of Lazurus is a helpful Gospel reading for a soul who has died this way, as well as all books and prayers of a spiritual nature. Ultimately, when the lessons are learned, they will move on to another realm of existence. They are cared for by loving spiritual helpers. Though at first so blinded with loneliness they cannot perceive such loving help, eventually they will realize the goodness in the universe and they can once again make a heartfelt choice for life.

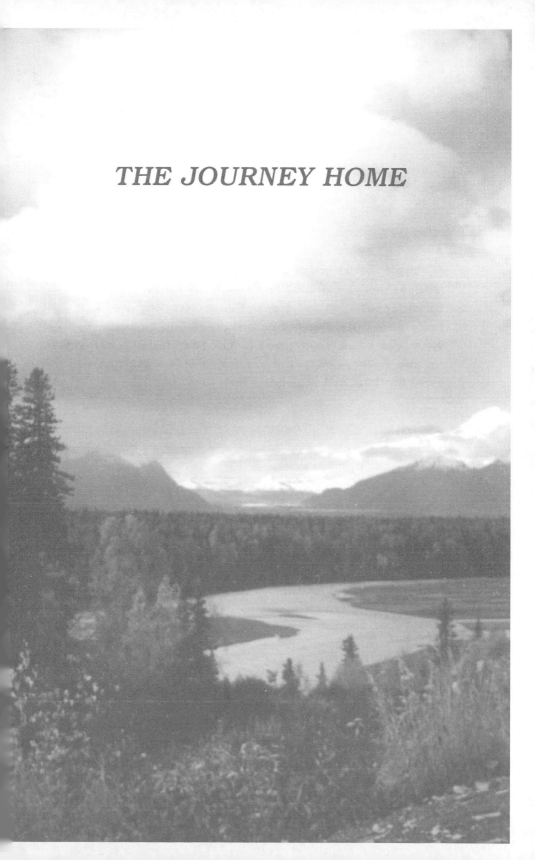

THE JOURNEY HOME

These stories speak of the journey "home" again and how the individual soul and spirit can be preparing for transition. The natural preparation for crossing over that takes place with aging is described, as well as how care-givers can support the process. The last stories are from the life journeys of two of our family elders and how we cared for them and celebrated their lives.

IS DESTINY ON COURSE?

Red didn't know he had cancer. The doctors didn't know it either until a month before he died. But when he called me to arrange a family reunion at our home, nearly a year before his transition, a sixth sense told me something was up. Red had married twice and never had a reunion with all his children or with his five siblings. He made sure this one was going to take place, and he worked it through all the diverse family channels with unwavering determination.

The gathering happened just the way he had hoped, laughter, jokes, food, hoopla and, above all, everyone just enjoying being together. Red was in a lot of pain by then, but he never spoke of it or let it show except that he didn't dance, standing by with a look of utter satisfaction on his face watching all the interactions and the family jubilee. When it was over, he had individually told everyone there that he loved them and had given each one of them a big bear hug in the process.

Red was a broad chested man with a deep sonorous voice, a shock of red hair, a broad go-to-hell grin, and a heart just as wide. The disease never noticeably wasted his strong body. Even near the end, he stepped from the shower in the buff and pulled a muscled stance for his wife and told her, "Check out this good looking guy!"

Already as a toddler Red heard a different drum, at the age of two following his own nose out into the streets of the sleepy little eastern Arizona town where he was raised. Shop keepers or neighbors would bring him home or telephone his family that he was wandering off again, but he never showed the least anxiety and merely waited for the next chance to go exploring on his own. He was going to follow his own star to the end.

Five days after the family reunion, the cancer was diagnosed and surgery prescribed for early the next week. The Sunday evening before, Red was outdoors in the hot tub, when a vision came to him of his long dead parents. They were young, happy and smiling, wanting to be with him. His mother came up and kissed him on the forehead and told him, "Red, everything is going to be all right." He came into the house jubilant. His pretty, brown-eyed wife, in her honeyed southern voice, described him as being in an altered state as he was telling about his vivid and unmistakable experience. He was elated and transformed, and thinking it could mean he would recover from the disease. She did not share his feelings, for all her senses spoke to a more sober reality. Yet she wondered at the powerful light and vitality around him.

On Monday he went to work, because in his ethic that was what men do. Tuesday morning he visited with one of his favorite nephews and his wife who had come to see him because they sensed his coming transition. But he was filled with optimism, and again enthusiastically shared the vision of his parents, and then went to the hospital for surgery.

He never left the hospital after the operation. A powerful man, it would take him awhile to leave his body. His beloved wife and son were at his side when he died three weeks later, taped, patched, tubed and coverless in the intensive care unit. But there wasn't going to be any long drawn-out lingering. His great heart had kept beating long enough for his warming grin to repeatedly push through the intense pain medication to tell everyone he was still on course and calling the shots as he basked in having all his family around the bed, praying and supporting him.

When Red had come to the reunion, and no one knew he was sick, he came to me and said in his no nonsense way, "Tell me what happens when you die." I was caught off guard. But I have never experienced such a candid look of intense and penetrating attention as I answered him. I gave him a picture of transition and how, once across, after a brief life review, we get to experience all the results of our actions in this life by experiencing the feelings of those who were effected by them.

He grinned and said, "Oh boy, I don't know about that!"

"Yes, some people call it hell," I countered, and we laughed. "But you get to experience all the good things you did, too," I added. I talked about the sharing and caring that goes on across the threshold.

Somewhere Red did know about his time of transition. His spirit made sure he had touched base with everyone before he left. It did work out "all right," as his parents who were waiting for him had promised.

When we listen to the stories of the last years or months of a person's life, many revealing threads come to light that often show there was a underlying fore-knowledge of the event. There can be quiet statements, plans to give away possessions, resolution of old angers or attachments. Messages of hope are often experienced that are given in the spiritual or eternal sense, and not necessarily an indication that recovery will be forthcoming on the physical plane. One woman during her long battle with cancer before her death, awoke from a deep sleep with a feeling of pressure on her shoulder and heard the words, "Everything will be all right" and felt an angel had spoken directly to her. She knew she was in higher hands.

History gives us the example of Joan of Arc, who had a fervent sense of her own destiny. Astride her great war horse, with fresh face and shining armor, grasping her sword that never killed a man, she cried, "I was born for this!" Thus she could give firm voice to her life's path, even though a fiery death awaited her after she had led French army to change the face of Europe.

A beautiful, popular young girl who died suddenly in a car accident had written in her journal only the month before, "I know what my mission in life is and why I have lived . . . to give love to others."

I urge people to pay attention to the events in the months, year, or even a few years before the death of a loved one to find the hints of their higher spiritual statements or intentions. Consider the people they met, the conversations they had, the closures they made, the last gifts they bestowed, the coming full circle of life, the final gifts. Often they have made journeys to old haunts and friends, written or called significant people in their lives, found ways to let us know that things are indeed, "going to be all right" in the bigger spiritual plan.

The parents of a five-year-old girl with leukemia had pursued every medical possibility to prolong her life and were shaken with her death. Yet with great devotion and gratitude, the child's mother was able to begin a spiritual communion with her daughter in the spiritual world, including a perspective on how her child's destiny had manifest in such a brief life on earth. She once conveyed a question to her heavenly child, "Emily, do you remember how it was when you were so sick and we were praying for a miracle?" Her spirit child sent back this answer, "Mother, you got a miracle. I am where I need to be, and I am always with you." Then she added with angelic wisdom, "It's all about love, Mother, and that never goes away."

MAKING A PLAN

It is most rewarding in this work to make funeral plans with someone who recognizes that they are actually going to die and then does something about it.

Doré was such a practical planner. Firm jawed, trim, with white hair cut in a no-nonsense bob, she was a remarkable survivor of life's dramas. She often said she felt she was cramming several lifetimes into one. She had been married and had two sons and a daughter. During her life she was challenged with alcoholism, abuse, divorce, cancer, and one son dead by his own hand. Through it all, she fearlessly forged on, shouldered the pain and wrote a book about the subject to help others. There was not an ounce of self-pity or sentimentality in her makeup. She had a blunt honesty that could border on the tactless, but she definitely cleared away the hyperbole and left you free to deal with the bare facts—or not deal with them.

In later life, when asked to write an autobiography, she sputtered, "I've spent seventy years being ashamed of my life and now I'm asked to write about it! But it's finally making sense!"

She had high blood pressure and an uneven heart beat that gave an urgency to her world travel, lecturing and promoting her book about her special connection to her son who had committed suicide. She had taken to heart the words of Rudolf Steiner, spiritual teacher and philosopher, who encourages the strengthening of the relationship with those across the threshold by reading for them. The reading can be from any books of eternal spiritual value through which one is to able to convey timeless ideas. The Bible, especially St. John, the Bhagavad-Gita, Shakespeare, poetry such as Wordsworth's, the soul's evolution as is portrayed in myth and fairy tales, Ralph Waldo Emerson, and Rudolf Steiner's spiritual science are all good resources. Conversely, the one in the spiritual world, not confined to a body, can offer broad and knowledgeable spiritual caring for the loved one left behind who has opened up this path of communication.

With dogged persistence, Doré read to her son day after day, month after month, year after year, following his death. Slowly she was able to experience his awakening from pain and isolation to greater enlightenment. Her energy, faith, and deeds aided in his birth to a new level of comprehension and awareness of his immortal existence. He aided her from the other side in writing a book to help many who have suffered through this tragedy of suicide.*

Once I asked Doré after she had spent some years counseling people who had experienced suicide in their families, if many of them came to her searching for solace and comfort. Her answer was instructive.

"I've learned, Nancy, that the spirit is not about comfort. The spirit takes you where you would not go. It's about growing and consciousness. It's the soul that wants comfort. But the truth is that the only way the soul can gain comfort is to take on the challenges it faces and overcome and transform them." Priceless wisdom from one who has faced the pain and has been tirelessly striving on the spiritual path.

Doré called me one day, determined to get all her own funeral arrangements in order.

"Number one is the doctor, Doré," I told her. "You have to be working with a physician in the event you have a home death. Legally in this state (and most others) you have to have seen a physician within a few weeks before the death for the doctor to be able to sign the death certificate as to the cause of death. If not, the authorities can, and usually do, require an autopsy to determine why the death occurred. You don't want an autopsy if you can avoid it. Get a doctor you can work with for a home death and tell him or her what you are planning."

We then went over the death and cremation certificates. With her typical ability to face things head on, she was going to the funeral home the next day to get all the information together for her own death certificate.

"You'll need your mother's maiden name and where your mother and father were born. They are also very particular about how the date is written. You'll need to supply an address where the ashes will be kept, at least for the time being," I told her.

We discussed having her vigil at the home of a good friend, as she felt her own apartment would not be suitable. Several times in the conversation, she interjected, "Now you'll have to be gentle with my children. They're not used to all this."

"It's not all that strange, Doré." I told her. "Many funeral situations have viewing as well as wakes and prayers for the dead. We've just added consciously reading or praying for the person throughout the day and night. But what do you want us to do for your son and daughter?" I asked her. "How do you see it happening? How can we support them? Since they live far away, will they need a place to stay here?"

"My daughter has in-laws here she can stay with," she said. "Of course, my children will have to deal with all my stuff."

"Then your son could stay in your apartment," I offered. She hesitated.

"Come on, Doré, of course he can stay there. You won't be there!"

When the obvious fact hit her, she howled with laughter, great long guffaws of mirth, after which she rejoined, "Nancy, you're a kick!"

So amidst serious directives and humor, we went over the plan, whom to call and what to arrange. She was left assured that she would get all the help and celebration the community could muster. It was a straightforward conversation in a style she understood. She was in charge and feeling good about it.

"Doré, you are really something and I love you," I told her as we finished.

"I love being here," she answered, and then added, "Rudolf Steiner says you stay connected with people you know when you cross over. You better think of me because I'm going to be in touch with you!"

It was my turn to laugh and I told her I didn't know of any conversation I'd ever had about planning for the transition that I had enjoyed more.

Light Beyond The Darkness, Doré Deverell

**Staying Connected,* Rudolf Steiner

A CONVERSATION ABOUT DYING

She was dying of cancer. Her daughters wanted to care for her at home and have a vigil to honor her when she died the way we had done in our community. They asked me to come and have a consultation with her. While her daughters had a spiritual view of life similar to my own, the mother did not. She was basically agnostic in outlook.

I met her on the back porch of her daughter's small pleasant home where she was living. She loved being outdoors to enjoy the day and spent as many hours there as her strength allowed. After we were introduced, her daughter left us and we began a conversation. She had been a school teacher in the inner city and had raised a large family alone. As a small child she had undergone traumatic experiences during the second World War. It had not been an easy life.

As she told me some things about her experiences, she smoked one cigarette after another with slender trembling hands. Though her daughter, understandably, was concerned about safety with her smoking, I gave her support for this comforting ritual. In chatting about her current situation she told me she got pretty crabby at times. I shrugged my shoulders and said that was a problem we all had to struggle with. We went on to talk about teaching, about people who could inspire the young, and touched on Martin Luther King, Jr. and Peace Pilgrim.

This was hardly the occasion for me (or anyone) to try to sway her views on life and death, or anything else for that matter. The point was how she felt about it. I asked her, "Pauline, how did you keep going all those years?"

She looked away. "Just a day at a time. I had a kind of faith that it was going to work out."

"So something was there you felt you could count on?"

"Yes."

The conversation went on and then, having gathered an impression of her approach to life, I ventured, "My sense is that you are someone who truly values freedom."

She turned her head abruptly, looking at me full on with sober, intense acknowledgement.

I lightly added, "I don't believe you want anyone to tell you what to believe."

She laughed and reached for another cigarette, and then went on to tell me some of the diverse views held by friends and family around her. Then her daughter and a grandson joined us. He was a favorite grandson, just twenty one, and he sat down close to her on the couch. It was clear they were devoted to each other. They told me how she had come to stay with him in his bachelor apartment and had met all his friends. He was obviously nervous at the prospect of talking about her dying.

I shared matter-of-factly the things we had done in our family, and what uplifting things can occur for everyone in the three days. Actually, Pauline was okay with the vigil idea. She had been thinking about the songs she wanted sung for the occasion. Her grandson didn't think he could handle being around the body. I tried to assure him that if he were able to be with her through her dying process, it would seem a natural part of it.

Even though Pauline didn't have a faith in life after death, it was interesting what followed. We somehow began talking about her father, whom she had loved and depended on, and greatly missed when he died. I asked when he had crossed over and when she told me, I noted it was only a few months after this favorite grandson had been born. It seemed natural to consider, in fact she even voiced it herself, that her father's caring for her was able to continue through this grandson who obviously had an unusually strong connection to her. "Sounds like that might have been a good plan to me," I offered. Something dawned for her as she considered this possibility.

Then they got everything on the table. She asked her grandson if he could handle her being gone, and he replied it would certainly be hard but he would manage. Then he turned to her and gently asked her, "Grandma, are you scared?" She told him, "No," and that she felt she could manage too. One felt them both relieved to have these concerns out in the open and brought into words. Her daughter turned to me and asked, "How are we doing?"

"I think you are awesome," I replied. "When three generations can talk about dying with such an open and significant sharing as this, it is truly a wonderful thing.

I had been there for nearly three hours. As I got up to leave, I looked at Pauline again. She was skeletal thin and fragile, but also translucent, transcendent...and beautiful. Tears came to my eyes as I told her so. "The body may be wasting away, but you can never take away the beauty of the spirit. This lady has a beautiful spirit," I told them.

She reached to take my hand and held it for a very long time. All the while, with a tiny smile at the corners of her mouth, she gazed at me with her blue eyes as wide, penetrating, and deep seeing as those of a small child when they drink in the world with unblinking intensity and openness. What an incredible look! At long last, I kissed her hand and we parted. As I left, as always, I felt gifted again with the magnificent wonder of the power of the human spirit at the threshold.

Post Script — As we had hoped, it turned out that it was her grandson and his fiancé who were holding Pauline's hands and reassuring her through her last hours and her passing. He also helped with her care and sang for her afterwards.

THE GRANDMA AND THE BABY

A grandmother of one of my students was visiting my nursery kinder-garten class. She sat on a kitchen chair amidst a circle of four and five-year-olds seated on smaller child-sized chairs. A tall woman, her large torso, bosom to hip, cascaded down in great amorphous slopes and her ankles swelled and overflowed the sensible shoes. On this day, like a story book grandma, she wore a cheerful yellow and blue apron, and a pale cardigan sweater stretched over her round shoulders. Her hands lay peacefully in her lap, age spotted, and worn from years of work. She smiled but said very little. Above the gravity weighted ballast of her grand old body, her face shone clear as the morning sun rising over solid rock mountains. Tendrils of white hair sprayed about her face like tiny etchings of an invisible halo. Her kindly countenance radiated blessing into the room, with eyes shining like jewels, bestowing wisdom-filled, compassionate light on all the children who sang, clapped and did their finger plays with round-eyed wonder and glee. Grandma's spirit abounded about her in clouds of goodness and voluminous warmth. Like contented kittens, the children basked in the golden benevolence of her presence.

Across the circle from her, I sat with my youngest child, a baby son, on my lap. His smooth pink cheeks were rose petal soft, the silken gold curls lay cradled in the sweet curve of the back of his neck. His chubby fingers were in constant motion, opening, closing, responding to the ripples of enthusiasm that ebbed and flowed through the group. But most of all, his dancing, innocent brown eyes were caught and held by the gaze and smile of Grandma. And she was held by him. The bond of their connection flowed on the invisible diameter of that circled group with a near tangible force. It was a connection that could hardly be missed, even by a casual observer.

"How attuned they are!" I marveled, "and actually at just about the same place."

It was true. The rosy, growing child was surrounded and made large by his spirit striving to get into his little body. A big spirit working to fit into a soft, flexible, chubby physical form, to flow out into the world, learning and growing into earthly life with each touch, sound, taste and smile. Grandma, her body fully lived through and worn with time, was preparing to leave it behind. Her spirit was now moving out, surrounding her as she was going back to the other side. Small boy part way in, dear old Grandma, part way out. One coming and one going!

They both knew it. They recognized each other like old colleagues that chummed with the angels on a regular basis, for each had one foot in the universe and one foot on earth. With knowing looks, they shared the levity, the secret of spirit existence in ways far transcending the often mundane experience of us mortals in the midst of life, whose identity can be so bound to our bodies. On a magical morning, in a wordless communion, the innocent babe and the gentle old grandma knew better.

See **PREPARING FOR THE JOURNEY**

THE FRUITS OF A LIFETIME

I have a friend and colleague I have worked with for many years. He is a scientist and a physician. For over a dozen years we have given seminars together on caring for the young child. As a research pediatrician, he has met and examined thousands of newborn babies, and, I am convinced, the world is better for it. I am confident those babies have become stronger individuals for having his kindly, compassionate and knowledgeable presence as one of their first sense impressions in life. He is a devout man and he is now a venerable elder in the community.

We have been a good team, working together to bring the spiritual, practical and scientific aspects of the care for the newborn and young child. Recently, we did another conference together. It has been my task to keep the timing in hand, managing question and answer sessions to fit in the necessary time allotted. But this time, as we were working to cover the predictable questions on infant issues, I found his answers expanding rather than condensing. At first I was frustrated, trying to figure out how to keep everything on track to finish on time. Then I realized the phenomena I was witnessing and my frustration was replaced with something of a sense of awe.

He was as sharp as ever, bringing a depth of knowledge in his field as he usually did. His meticulous devotion to scientific clarity and objectivity was as resonant as ever. There was no question of his capacities. But each question would trigger an entire lifetime of experience and knowledge. It was like a grand old apple tree, abundant with the finest ripe fruit. He willingly brought the harvest down to offer the group, not just one fruit but many, and on any subject that was brought up.

Linear time, going to a certain point and condensing the subject, was no longer the important thing for him. He was expanded. One felt the fruits of his lifetime of work filling the space around him, surrounding him. He could go anywhere. He could give the history, the researchers, the development of medical practices involved in the fullest detail. He was a man and his work in full bloom.

"This is just the time he should be mentoring younger physicians," I thought to myself. When I brought it up to him, I was most pleased to find that was exactly what was taking place.

This is just what needs to happen. Those who are striving in any work or profession should seek out those elders who can enrich their work. Such respect allows the gifts of a life to flow back into community life. It allows the legacy to be given. The elders will not respond in terse sound bytes. They are moving into richer and broader realms. Probably the fact that they are not of the computer generation can also make their experience and contributions all the more valuable as a legacy of balance in a highly technological society.

What a gift for everyone involved when someone can come and share the bounty of a lifetime of experience. Countless people have been enriched in recent years because a man was inspired to travel by plane every week to visit his old college professor who was dying of cancer. Because of this man's attentiveness, his faithfulness to bear to witness to the story, and to receive the wisdom from his teacher, *Tuesdays with Morrie,* the book about their sharing, came into existence. The world is richer for it.

My friend, the physician has become a wise elder of his profession. He is sharing the fruits of a lifetime, generously given to all those who are able to recognize and appreciate the gift as he travels his journey toward transition.

*See **PREPARING FOR THE JOURNEY***

NELLIE

Oh, Nellie, what a lady! On second thought maybe "grand old gal" would come closer to describing her. Her own proud self-description was even earthier, "wild old broad." She made her debut in a log cabin in New Mexico in 1902, lived ninety-two years, and, though she died in a nursing home, her funeral celebration was held on a cattle ranch in the Sierra Nevada between two great gnarled oak trees with her great-grand nieces sending balloons up into the last rays of flaming red sunset.

Nellie was the baby of a family of five. A cherubic charmer with gorgeous brown eyes, Nellie was adorable, willful, petulant and spoiled. She was born of earnest, sociable, hard-working pioneer folk of the time. Her mother was warm with a Southern woman's ways, and her father was destined to die young, when Nellie was only three. Her mother remarried a kindly Swedish immigrant they called Pappa Hollem, who was brave enough to take on the five young children along with the charming widow. Nellie was only eleven when her mother died also.

Bereft of both parents, Nellie refused to pity herself as an abandoned child. Rather, alone on a windswept night under a New Mexico moon, the gutsy, determined girl vowed that no one owed her anything, and, if she wanted something in life, she would darn well get it for herself.

Nellie had a sensuous love of life. Her soul filled with delight in the western skies and the purple mountains shimmering across the Western plains that she would later try to capture in paintings. She loved the smell of freshly cut wood, baking bread, wild flowers, and the grace of beautiful objects. She delighted in the furry warmth of dogs (she was never without one), deep fried chicken, and indeed every kind of good food. ("I was always hungry, honey," she'd declare.) When she grew up, she embraced life with zest, which included glamorous clothes in the latest classic style, dancing, a good cigarette, an occasional tart Marguerita, sex and, above all, the dynamic of fun and good times and conversation with all kinds of people. With little more than a grade school education, she was, nonetheless, by her own claim, "Good at everything I tried." She loved good hard work, and pitted her raw-boned strength against any job to be done. She took unabashed pride in transforming a place and making it shine.

When Nellie was fourteen, her Aunt Neen, a socialist party member and suffragette, felt responsible for her sister's orphans, and mounted an expe-

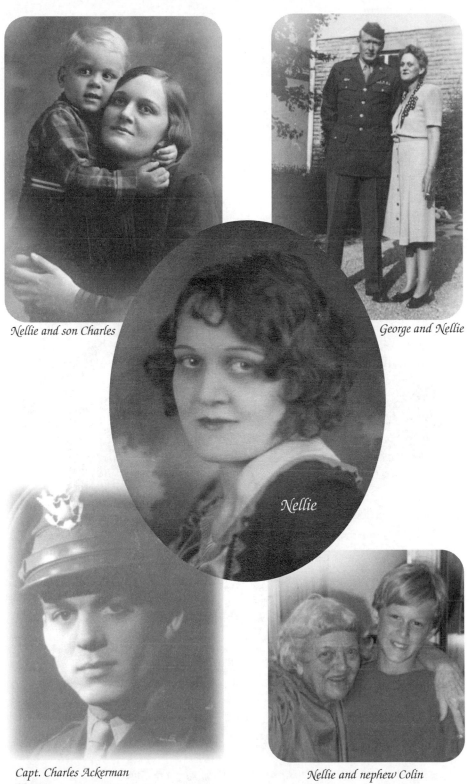

Nellie and son Charles

George and Nellie

Nellie

Capt. Charles Ackerman
23 years

Nellie and nephew Colin

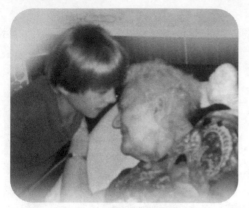
My grandson Alex visits Nellie

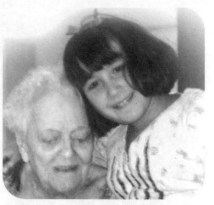
Nellie and my granddaughter Gabrielle

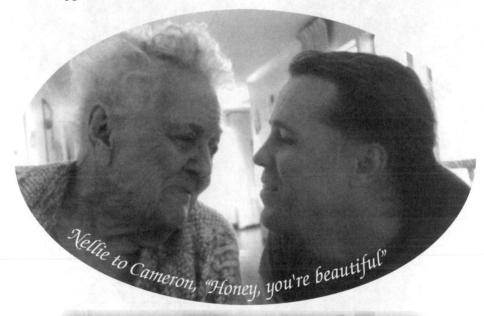
Nellie to Cameron, "Honey, you're beautiful"

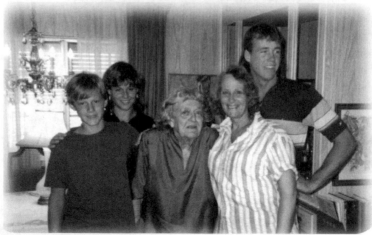
Nellie's Crew: Colin, Mary, Nancy & Cameron

dition to bring the families to a Utopian commune experiment in the deserts of California. Nellie loved it all: the community life, the work, the food, the music and especially the dances. She'd been dancing since she was five years old and knew all the moves from the days of community shindigs in New Mexico where Mexican virtuosos with dazzling skill played violins on Saturday nights at the old adobe dance hall, and where, on a nearby tree, the initials of Billy the Kid were carved

A few years later, along with her sister and cousins, Nellie went to Los Angeles and worked for Western Union as a switch board operator. There the girls once went out dancing for thirty nights in a row. Fox trot, Charleston, waltzes, they knew them all and they danced far into the night to live music in great cavernous dance halls with wonderful hardwood spring floors. It was prohibition time and bouncers, tough beefy men, guarded the doors to throw out anyone who drank or bothered the ladies. The open, good looking Western girls rarely sat out a dance, and they loved it.

It was his shoes, black patent leather and polished to a gleam, that first attracted Nellie. Then her eyes rose to the rugged, handsome face and the smooth-talking charm of the fancy dancing man, a divorced salesman thirteen years her senior. What a glamorous pair they made as they whirled around the dance floor! Nellie, the nineteen-year-old country girl, couldn't resist his polished advances, and a fast courtship and marriage quickly followed. But soon after, when Nellie was in full bloom with child, Mr. Patent Leather Shoes was long gone.

In a little flat at the end of the street-car line in Redlands, feisty Aunt Neen and Nellie's goggle eyed sister, Lola, attended her as she went into labor for the birth. Nellie gave enormous announcement to the world of the coming event. With her typical gusto, she didn't even try to hold back. Her screams, raising in volume with each labor pain, echoed throughout the neighborhood until the poor street-car driver cringed to drive his passengers by as he went on his route up and down the street. After the big, lusty boy, Charles, was born, Nellie received baby gifts not only from trolley passengers, but from sympathetic strangers for blocks around as well. Already, one way or another, Nellie was taking care of her own. As she nursed her own handsome son, she wet-nursed a fragile baby girl to health at the same time, gaining the everlasting gratitude of the child's parents.

Nellie and her son had an extraordinarily close relationship. They cared for each other and shared artistic gifts; painting, a love of drama, and common courage for the full cup of life. When Charles was three, Nellie married a tough, courageous, but unsympathetic Air Corps pilot. A few years later she watched the little boy born of that union die a painful death from meningitis as she stood helplessly by, separated from her young child who lay quarantined and dying behind thick hospital glass. The marriage came apart.

Nellie worked as a waitress, raised her only son, and kept a spotless house. Having few luxuries in her youth, she took joy and pride in her home. During World War II, she met her life long love: a tall, gangly, handsome, ruddy-faced Georgia man with a thatch of curly white blond hair. Taking the shy, inexperienced young man in hand, she introduced him to love making in a California orange grove. Theirs would be a faithful union lasting nearly fifty years. An Air Corps sergeant and mechanic, her husband served long years in the toughest war theaters, brooded over the planes he repaired for war, and prayed for their crews. Nellie's son, Charles, became an Air Force pilot, and, after fifty wartime missions, twice the usual combat tour of duty, he crashed into a fog shrouded mountain in a B-17 and died with a crew of comrades. He was twenty-three.

Nellie screamed with a broken heart and inconsolable grief. Then, never passive in the face of pain, she scrubbed every square inch of the house from attic to basement and thereafter poured out the fierce love of her big passionate heart on all her nieces and nephews and the other young men from Charles' Air Force squadron

We always loved our Aunt Nellie when we were growing up. We admired her beautifully kept home, and were fascinated with her glamorously painted nails and makeup, her elegant clothes, the languorous roll of her cigarette, and the wild charm of her stories. Wherever Nellie was, there was fun and laughter. And Nellie enjoyed us. She warmly supported our lives, loves and accomplishments. Even though she occasionally swore and called herself a "heller," she couldn't fool us. We knew her courage and human goodness went bone deep. Nellie refused to be bitter about the great sorrows she had endured. She continued to love the beauty of the world and everything in it, especially young people, her garden, her painting, and her beloved husband. Her unwavering spiritual faith was expressed daily in Unity prayers, which she always shared with us as her faithful witness to the Lord's goodness.

In old age, after a failed surgery on her knee, Nellie was confined to nursing homes where she would live out the last several years of her life. Always a storyteller given to vivid and exaggerated tales, her imagination only became more animated with age. Intermittent dementia added novel twists to the tales. Her inner world grew more vivid and increasingly peopled with marvelous characters such as Big Red, her faithful Persian helper, bevies of animals, great German shepherds, fairy coaches pulled by precious miniature horses or elegant butterflies, and a ten-foot rattlesnake named Hank who was "really friendly and could stand on his tail." When I inquired one day about Hank's whereabouts, she told me he'd gone down to Palm Springs for the weekend. She regularly assured me she was famous since she was daily making records in the recording studios which were going to bring in millions to take care of everyone in the whole family. Once when I asked her what the songs she sang were about, she paused and looked at me with those wonderful brown eyes and said, "Oh, honey, just about all of the joys and sorrows of life."

The wanderings of her mind were the despair of her gentle, rational husband. He confided to me he didn't feel he had long to live, and he was touchingly grateful when I told him our family would look after Nellie if he went first. He was right. He died soon after, and we prepared for the great journey from half a state away to bring Nellie to a home near us. As she was afraid of flying, we equipped the van with the softest mattress we could find and planned an all-night transport. My son, Cameron, and daughter, Mary, completed the team. Though one of us always lay beside her for comfort and fed her grapes or anything she asked for, she declared repeatedly we were trying to kill her on the rough roads. When we lamely tried to explain we were going by car because she didn't want to fly, she ordered us to stop and said she would "buy the goddamned airport and an airplane" so she could "darn well get there sooner!" It was a long trip.

However, Nellie slept some even if we didn't and when we pulled into a drive-in for breakfast, bleary eyed and exhausted, she perked up and asked for breakfast "with eggs, hash browns all the fixin's" which she ate with gusto. Then we went to the nursing home.

As she was lowered into a bed, Nellie reached up to give her attendant a soft touch on the cheek and with a big smile, delivered the endearing greeting she always gave everyone. In her gravelly voice, raspy from years of smoking, she said, "Honey, you're beautiful." But the mood didn't last.

In this nursing home, there was no special sympathy for her charm, except from one open young girl. Nellie was angry. She swore. She threw food. She wheeled herself along the halls and stole milk off the food carts, she spit on the floor, and worse. The hospital director was ex-army and wanted the place in top military order. One day as the facilities were being inspected by authorities from the state, Nellie pulled off her night gown as they came down the hall, sat stark naked in her wheelchair and defiantly stared them down. Against our wishes, the management put her on heavy psychotropic drugs. These only drove her further into rebellion.

I was called to a tribunal. I walked into a room filled with a staff of eight sitting stony faced around a long conference table. I had hoped to plead Nellie's case but was met with an immovable wall of cold antipathy. No one wanted to work with her there and, furthermore, they wanted her "out of here—now!" It was harsh.

I couldn't believe it. "Wait a minute," I thought. "She's on state aid. You can't kick a ninety-year-old lady out of a facility with no place to go!" They could, and they would. Angrily, I pleaded for time and began frantically searching for another home. Good grief, she's an old woman pushing a century in years and kicked out like a delinquent! I was desperate. I pulled out the yellow pages of the telephone book and systematically phoned every facility in the big city. No one had state Medi-Cal beds available. Finally one kind administrator's voice gave me some hope. As I walked into that nursing home and looked down the halls, I was struck by the multi-ethnic staff: Filipino, Black, Hispanic, Asian and newly arrived Russian immigrants. Warm hued faces, compassionate brown eyes and ready smiles met me. Hope sprang up.

"Nellie," I thought to myself, "I think you're home." Needless to say, I didn't give the head nurse any more details than she needed.

I stayed with Nellie from morning to night for the next three days, mediating between her and the staff. I made sure she didn't throw food and let them know what a warm, funny and caring person she really was. A Filipino man, Napoleon, was her main caregiver. I showed my appreciation to him in every way I could, and held my breath in hope it would work. Napoleon's compassion ran deep as it did in other staff members; they didn't run to a head nurse with her every infraction but gave Nellie some leeway. Warm, good, tolerant people, this was what she needed and she responded to them. They became fond of her and this would become, for nearly two years, her last home.

Family members came as often as any of us could. We sang for her, brought flowers and treats, polished her nails and fixed her hair, gave her foot rubs, and had friends do eurythmy, a special movement therapy, for her. We made sure she always had Snooper, the stuffed dog she cherished for companionship, beside her pillow.

I sensed there was a wisdom in these years for Nellie. For one who had lived as deeply into the sensuous pleasures as she had, these years were a time of letting go of the physical drives and impulses little by little. It was a time of giving up strong attachments to the earthly senses, of becoming less encumbered with desires. I felt she would have fewer physical urges to purge and transform on the other side when she got there. Though her spirit never faded, she gradually released her grip on the earthly, and spiritually she became lighter and freer as the time came closer to leave her body.

The administration of the nursing home knew I wanted to bring her home to die with us. But Nellie fooled us all. She seemed sweet and faraway when I last saw her. Two days later, in the middle of the night they called me to say she seemed to be close to dying. Hearing the description of her symptoms, I debated whether or not to wait until morning. Then in my mind's eye her sister, Lola, my mother, came to me. She had died years before, but now with the enthusiasm of a cheer leader, she was urging me to "Go, go, go!" I climbed into the car at one o'clock in the morning for an hour's drive.

Nellie was in a light coma when I arrived, a blessing because she had always been so afraid of choking when she began to cough, and the coma overrode such choking. They told me she couldn't hear me. I knew better. I leaned close to her ear and whispered, "Nellie, I'm here." I felt her respond.*

Her breathing was deep, slow, and regular. I felt her body. It was warm. I wondered if she was really going now. I stayed by her with quiet prayers, and encouragement. The attendant came and took her blood pressure. I felt her legs, belly and face. Cold, then warm, then cold again. I could follow the effect of the rising and falling blood pressure readings in the warmth and cold of her body. Nellie was in labor for her spiritual birth. Her efforts were long, steady and productive. The process was just as rhythmic as that of birthing a child. The spirit moved part way out with a push, then back in, then expanded again with another push. The periodic blood pressure readings gave me another affirmation of the labor process, but as the night waned, I became exasperated with this interference in her process and finally told the aide, "Leave her alone, she's dying."

I sang to her. She loved singing, and she had loved Christmas. Nobody celebrated Christmas with more joy than Nellie. One of her earliest memories, that she had shared with me many times, was of her mother climbing a ladder to light the candles on top of their tall, fragrant Christmas tree, fresh from the New Mexico forest. No matter how poor they were, they always had a big tree. Her dear mother, whom she had known so briefly ("Who you would love, honey, and she would love you") would make each Christmas a magical one.

So though it was autumn, I sang Christmas songs for her, for it was Nellie's time for her Christmas birth into spirit. I sang *Oh, Holy Night.* It was amazing how the words fit for her crossing. *"Fall on your knees, Oh, hear the Angel voices, Oh, night divine, Oh, night when Christ was born."* Oh, night when you shall be born, dear Nellie, and be with the loving Savior.

Dawn streaked the sky. I had called the priest. He came with the communion, the holy words, the tiny crumb on her tongue, a tiny drop of consecrated grape juice. Her pace of breathing decreased, but never wavered in its steady determination. Then, just before she breathed her last, the great brown eyes opened wide with wonder and astonishment as she looked across into the spiritual world she would now enter. "Godspeed, Nellie, we love you." It was good.

It was good, but the setting was terrible. Four times in the process I had to turn off the television blaring across the room, which no one was watching. Every time I turned it off, someone would turn it on again. The hall banged with mop buckets and breakfast trays. As in most nursing homes, there was no sacred space for family, no time or place for any of the aides who had so patiently cared for her, feeding and bathing her through the days and years, to come bid their farewell and make closure. The inhumanity of it left me angry and saddened for all concerned. There was no way to have the room hallowed and sacred, except through her deed of dying. I had to get out of there. I had called the children, Lauren and Cameron, and they arrived just after she crossed over.

I was determined to take her home where we had her casket all in readiness. I told the head nurse and asked for a gurney. They didn't have one. "You can't do this," she told me, never having dealt with anyone other than a mortician to take the body away.

"Oh, yes I can," I replied. "She died here of natural causes. The doctor will sign the death certificate, and I am the next of kin who has the right to disposal of the body." Technically, I should have waited until the county offices were open, chased down the doctor to sign the death certificate, taken it to the county for filing, gotten the proper papers and then moved her, but that would have taken hours or even a day or more. Ironically, any funeral home attendant can take away the body at any time. What I did was not the technically legal process to begin with, though all the legal work was in place in the end.

I simply knew I had to get her out of there and away from the insane call bells, clanging mop buckets and blaring televisions. As there was no gurney, I looked up at my tall six-foot-five-inch son who was standing with a look of quiet love for Nellie on his handsome face. My daughter Lauren wore the same expression. "You game?" I queried. "You bet!" he replied.

So with infinite gentleness, Cameron lifted her body into his powerful arms as Lauren and I arranged a sheet over it. Then he carried his burden reverently into the hall and out the back door to his waiting truck, a pickup with a camper shell. Clusters of aides in the hall gasped and held their hands to their mouths as we paraded out. They had never seen anything like it. Later in the day, I would get the legal work tidied up. But for now we were out of there. (A week later I would take a huge box of chocolates for all the nursing home staff as a gift from Nellie).

In our home we laid her on the couch. Lauren, my eldest daughter, helped me bathe and dress her. (This was my daughter who, as an adolescent, adamantly wanted nothing to do with "Mama and the dead people!" After this experience she would find herself giving invaluable support to many others at death.) Together we placed Nellie's body in the beautiful casket Cameron had made. We draped a rich violet cloth over the window behind the casket and placed paintings by her and her son Charles around it. She looked elegant, and she was smiling.

It was near Halloween. My eight-year-old grandson set about purposefully, all on his own, to make his Halloween jack-o-lantern, carefully carving out the word "LOVE" to be illuminated from within. He set it down with quiet devotion beside the casket. Ten-year-old Gabrielle brought flowers and sweetly placed them in Nellie's hair. We sang, we read, we prayed, remembered, celebrated and decided the final funeral service should be out in the woods.

So it came to be that after the three days, friends loaded her casket onto the old 1927 Dodge Graham truck that had been in the family for over sixty years. The kids had festooned it with crepe paper streamers and balloons. Wally, the Dalmatian dog, stood nearby at attention. A dog to the very end for Nellie. I have a memorable picture of my grandson and me sitting with the casket on the back of the truck as it headed down into the woods, with balloons popping as it went through the trees. "Hooray! Nellie's, going out with a bang!" we all said.

We gathered family, friends and children on benches among the trees. The sun was setting. There was something so elegant, so amazingly unique, so profoundly artistic and beautiful about the whole thing: the soft light wood of the casket with its elegant sculptured handles; the deep turquoise cloth on the table beneath it, bordered with a gleaming yellow row of sun-warm marigolds from the garden; son Cameron, standing in tall dignity in his black and white robes as he assisted the minister, also a big and impressive man robed in similar somber vestments. It was all like a Rennaisance painting against the background beauty of the forest. The great gnarled oaks that framed the casket were like pillars of a cathedral, the cathedral Nellie loved most of all, the perfect beauty of the church of nature. She was blessed and honored, I told her life story. We played music and sang, *"Swing low sweet chariot, comin' for to carry me home."* Later, Cameron would take the final journey to the crematorium.

Dear Nellie, how your zest for life rings through your stories today, and while you left no children of your own on the planet, you left the vibrantly living legacy of your gift of fun, joy and universal love for all the world and everything in it. Godspeed, beloved Nellie!

*See **COMA**

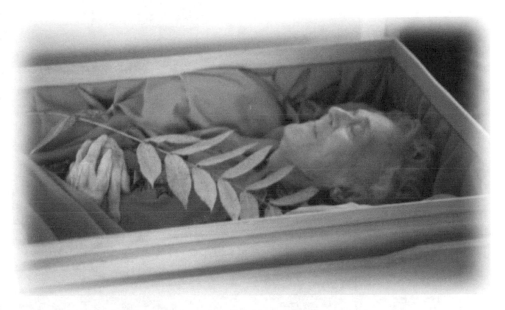

Nellie at Peace

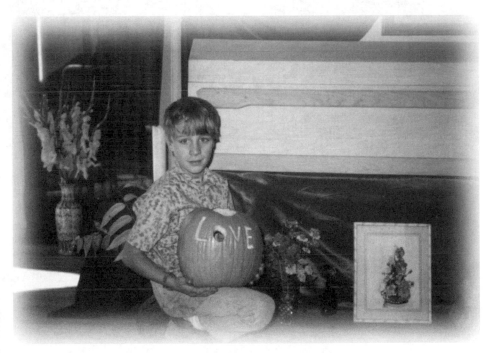

Alex with his pumpkin of love for Nellie

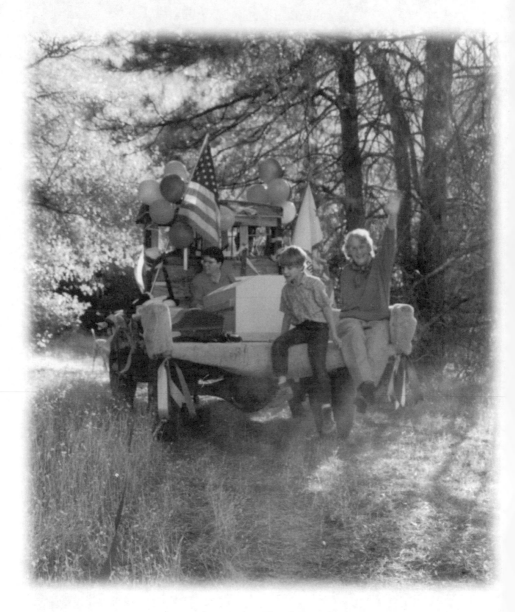

Our Farewell to Nellie

PAPPY

When I began writing this book I hadn't expected to share my father's story, but I've found it includes experiences I hope may be helpful to others. Pappy was the name given to my father by his oldest grandchild and it stayed with him the rest of his life. He taught me about life, and no less profoundly he taught me through his death. At the end of his life he was a fully bedridden invalid, and my husband left his profession for nearly two years to care for him, just as I had cared for my husband's grandmother, Mary Edna.

I was impressed by the grace of my father's passing. There was an underlying endurance, a sense of pacing himself to do what he had to do. He was a man with a plan. It is hard to imagine how a man so fully engaged in life, a teacher of men and boys with the keenest of minds and the ability to deftly translate ideas into physical reality; a man who was felling huge pine trees in his seventies, jogging into his eighties and still dancing in his nineties, could come to passive immobility with such equilibrium. He almost never complained.

First of all, I learned that his helpless condition did not detract one whit from who he really was. He was no less a man, no less my beloved father as he lay helpless in a hospital bed, than he had been all my life. Many people avoid seeing people they know when they have lost their earthly prime. True, it can be a shock. But, if one is trying to sense the spiritual aspect of the situation, it becomes another truth. Pappy had been born in the nineteenth century. He grew up with no pollution, with unprocessed, healthy food, with hard work and exercise and none of the wasting aspects of modern life. He was tough. And he was well integrated into the physical. It was going to take a process to chip the spirit out of that wiry, old, fully used body. It took a heart attack, two strokes, and a year and half of loosening up and letting go before he was ready.

When he had his stroke, I immediately flew down to his home to be with him. His wife of over fifty years had died two years before, leaving him alternately bewildered, lonely, sad and angry. Now with the stroke, he was half blind and, as I met him, he handed me his wallet with a brusque command, "Here, you take care of this." "Giving up his power," one could think, but instead I sensed a great relief behind his words. He had always taken care of the money. Now he would no longer, ever again, have to worry about finances.

I went outside the house to look at what would prove to be the last creative act he was able to perform on earth out of his own initiative. His home was in a Southern California town by the ocean. A large, exotic tropical vine called Cup-of-Gold grew across the western side of the house. It had huge, bowl shaped blossoms with delicately curled edges, some up to a foot across. The vine had been neglected, and long runners streamed across the ground. Pappy set out to take care of the problem but, instead of securing the stray vines to the trellis along the house, he got a stake and put it out in the middle of the lawn. Then he got on a ladder and nailed a makeshift piece of wood from the top of the stake to the house. He tied the vine up with string so it was running out perpendicular from the house and towards the ocean. The great, golden blossom was open to the West, like a Grail cup waiting to receive and be filled with the shining light of the setting sun. As I later looked back on this, his last deed, I was moved and impressed.

I took him to see the doctor, a specialist. I drove the car to a parking place by the clinic and got out and went around to take him by the arm and guide him over the curb. He had dressed carefully, in a blue shirt, a checkered sports coat and slacks, and a smart tie. He was a handsome man with black curly hair now salt and pepper gray. He took my arm, and we walked down the sidewalk together. It was late afternoon, the sunlight slanted through the leaves of the trees; clouds came scudding in from the seashore, and there was a salty tang in the air. It was then, proud and erect, he pronounced the indelible words that have never left me.

"I think things are working out just about right."

"Just about right?" I thought to myself, "Sure, your wife died, you had a stroke and you are nearly blind. You can't drive a car or handle your own finances any more. Just about right?" However, he was grinning his I've-got-the-answer grin and getting ready to jest and show off with the doctor's receptionist.

As I waited during his consultation with the doctor, it dawned on me what I had just witnessed as we had entered the clinic. Here was a man with an astonishing sense of his own destiny. His spiritual self was coming through the words and declaring that, despite all outer appearances, destiny was right on track. Amazing! When a person's voice has that "pay attention" edge to it, when a statement seems to drop in from another plane of awareness, one senses this can be the higher self, imbued with spiritual knowing, sounding through ordinary daily consciousness. The old man was still in charge.

Many people in the community came to visit him after he became an invalid. He had a beautiful, old antique music box that played *The Blue Danube.* It was in his room by his bed, and the children loved to put thick, old English pennies in the slot to begin the whirl of the disks and dance to the sweet tinkling melody. One day a blonde, cherub-faced three-year-old girl came and did a dance, crawled on Pappy's bed, and patted his hand. But Pappy never said a word, he just lay looking into space with a glance or two at the child. Yet when mother and child stood at the door waving goodbye, he said in the most kindly and appreciative voice, "It gives me the greatest pleasure when you young people come to visit me."

It takes energy to die. Sometimes the old ones and the very ill cannot muster the will to enter into daily conversation. Like an ancient hermit huddled by a small, warm stove in the kitchen of a big, old, ever more dilapidated house, it is often just too much effort to leave that inner place of preoccupation and quiet to go down a long, drafty hall to the front door to greet someone out there with small talk.

Pappy's mind wandered. A life-long teacher, the ramblings were usually about working on projects for the young people. He always wanted to be sure they were getting opportunities to develop themselves. He always said that every youngster ought to be able to play a musical instrument and know a poem to recite "whenever the occasion called for it." By example, he often vigorously recited for us Robert Service poems, especially *The Shooting of Dan McGrew.*

One day we took him out to the back yard in his wheel chair to soak up sun and nature scents and to be with the dog. Grasping the arm rests of the chair, he sat bolt upright and suddenly made a declaration in his most imposing oratory. He bellowed out this gem of a legacy . . . a maxim that just about covers it all:

"If you can't laugh, don't get in line!"

In other words, he was telling us, "Don't bother to come down to be born, because, for sure, if you can't laugh you're going to have a heck of a time lining up for the dramas of life, much less crossing back to the other side." It was some of the best advice he ever gave us.

Only once did he berate me during his long confinement in our home when he said that he wanted "someone to get me out of here now, and I don't want just a bunch of drones to do it either!"

"Well, Pappy," I countered, "that's up to you. You're the one who sets the timing. William Blake says the door of death is covered with gold. That means the sun will be shining in front of your star when it's the time to go home. The moon stood in front your star when you came down to be born. The baby determines the time it wants to be born, too, and starts the labor for the birth."

"Well, that's interesting," he replied, "Tell me more."

And so I did. I told him how he needed just the right time to re-enter the spiritual world and give the fruits and gifts of his lifetime back into the universal good; how his loved ones would be waiting for him; how he would have work over there with like minded spirits; how he would have a life review and go through a catharsis; how he would look over our tasks on earth and send us love and ideas and support; and how our love would always be there for each other and the threshold would be no barrier to it. This was pretty much the one and only in-depth spiritual conversation we had. But the restless demands were gone. He seemed to settle into his work of moving on with the same enduring perseverance and resolve he'd applied to life for over nine decades.

One day I walked into his room and sat on the extra bed where we often slept to be there with him when needed. I was preparing my lessons for teaching that day. It was a glorious morning. Bright sunlight streamed through the sheer pink curtains and filled the room with a rosy glow. On the wall behind his bed was a beautiful painting of the Pieta (Mary holding the crucified Christ) in rich flowing colors. From where he lay, he could look at a large, beautiful print of a mother and infant child by Raphael. Both themes, new birth and death, are often found in ancient churches at the doors where one enters and leaves the building, the thresholds of coming and going, of birth and death. There were fresh flowers and a candle nearby. He lay curled in a fetal position staring into space. He inquired gruffly as I entered, "Who's that?"

"It's your daughter, Pappy," I laughed. He laughed back as I kissed him, and he gave me that mischievous Tom Sawyer grin of his. I sat on the bed. These were glorious moments. Here was my father, totally helpless as a babe lying in a hospital bed. But what mattered, the only thing that really mattered then and in the whole scheme of things, was that we loved each other. That love flowed in and around us and filled the room. It flowed out the windows and into that glorious morning sunshine and into life with a permeating warmth that nothing could stop, ever. We both knew it and that sharing still makes me smile, these many years later, every time I think of it.

His death was quiet and good though we had to go through some medical drama beforehand. He had a serious infection, and we took him to the hospital for an assessment. Had he stayed there, he would have been full of tubes and hooked to machines. He was too weak to speak by now. I took his hand in mine, and he gave my hand the strongest squeeze he could muster, though the touch of his fingers was scarcely perceptible. Yet with that faint and delicate sign, I knew he was saying vehemently, "Don't leave me here!" My dear husband agreed to take the intense nursing task on, and we took him back home.

He lay quietly on the bed back in the familiar room. His hands, once callous with work, had come back full circle, and were again as soft and tender as a young child. The body, thin and fully used, was spent. He was ready to go. We sang with him, sat and held his hand and massaged him when it seemed to give comfort. We gave him tiny sips of fluid when he needed them. The youngest grandchild, ten-year-old Colin, bounced in the room from playing with the dog outside his window and cheerfully said, "Have a good time in heaven, Pappy. We love you!" We had last rites and took shifts reading and praying with him. But he was still in charge for the time of actually going. As my husband lay sleeping near him in the room, he marched across the threshold to his own tune. Then the wind suddenly blew through the house slamming my bedroom door at three in the morning and I raced down the stairs to his room. He had just gone. "So like his style," I thought between feelings of awe, sorrow, and admiration.

What I now relate is so far beyond the bounds of ordinary perspective that it is difficult to believe. But it is a slice from life in all its real spiritual vibrancy.

My father's death and the accompanying three-day vigil at home gave many families in our community the opportunity to give their children an experience of death in a healthy, natural family setting. People streamed in and out of the room where he lay in light-filled space. The sun shone through the sheer rosy curtains on the cheerful flowers and mementos around the open casket. His presence was strong even in death. His chiseled countenance gave the impression of an old battle-worn but triumphant knight laid in final rest.

A family with a six-year-old boy came. The father, a teacher, sat in the room with the child on his lap and read aloud a story about a young boy who loved life and the world. Amidst the general bustle in the household, I noticed how happy and excited the boy seemed. For some reason the family decided to return the following evening to continue the vigil and read more of the story for the child. I again noticed, how eager the child was, his face aglow in the candlelight.

I was not often in touch with the family as the boy grew up, and they moved away to another state. Twenty years later, I chanced to stay with the parents while giving lectures for a conference in their town. While I was there, their son, now a young adult, called home. His mother told him I was there and then to identify me, explained that I was Pappy's daughter. Her son responded in a voice filled with delight. The mother's statement apparently stirred a long forgotten childhood memory of a treasured old friend. "Pappy!" he exclaimed with enthusiasm.

Why is this so amazing? Because he and Pappy never actually met each other in physical life! They met at the threshold of death, after Pappy "died." And what a meeting it was! The child, young, innocent, receptive and open, could experience the outpouring of vitality of Pappy's ninety two years of living, his soul and spirit essence filling the space where they met with the substance of a long life and a career devoted to the development of young people, especially boys. Pure communion. Spirit to spirit!

The warmth of that meeting radiated into the life of that young man from then on. Here through the lasting experience of a child, we can grasp the incredible gifts which can flow into the broader community of life when we can come to the threshold with open, supportive awareness. Everyone is blessed.

Lola and Oren (Pappy)

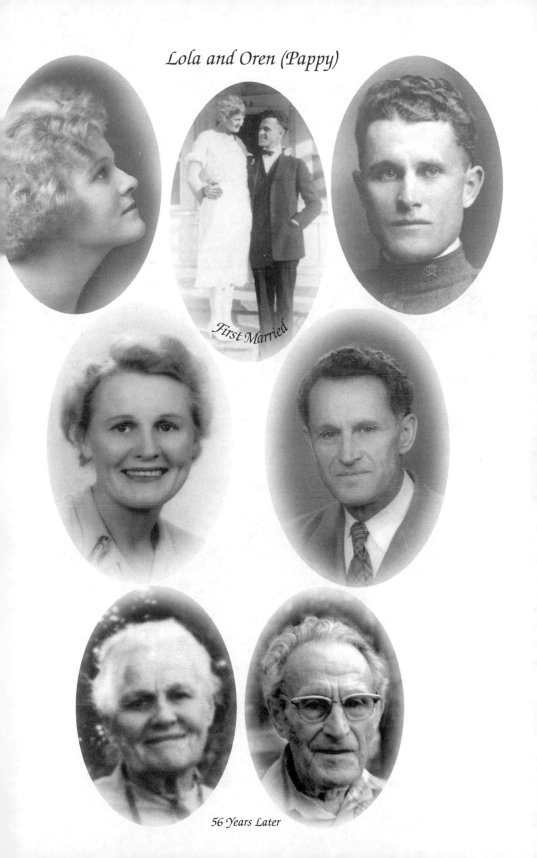

First Married

56 Years Later

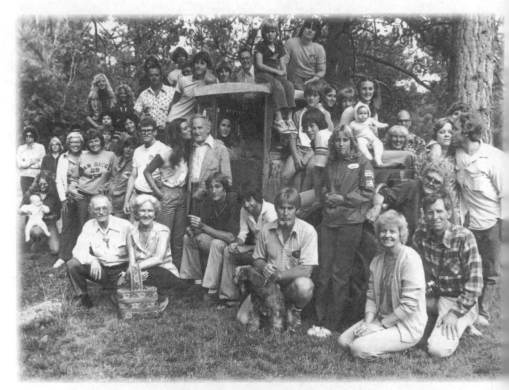

Pappy's 90th Birthday

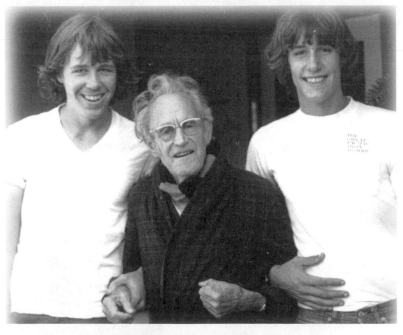

Pappy with Grandsons Cameron & Gary

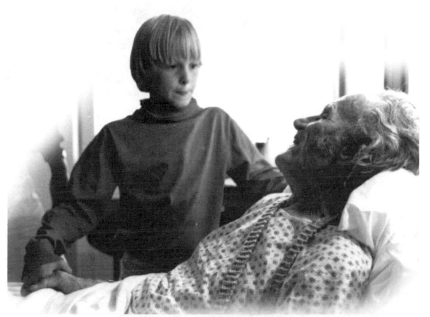

Colin & Pappy on his 91st birthday

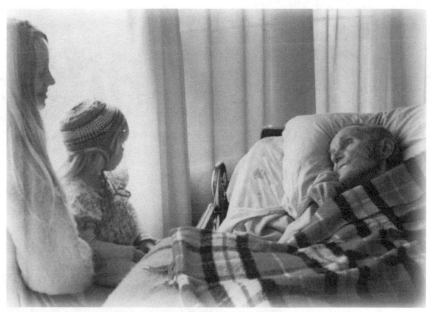

"It gives me the greatest pleasure when you young people come to visit me."

Pappy had a 1927-Dodge-Graham truck at the ranch. He kept it running for over fifty years and gave rides to generations of family and friends.

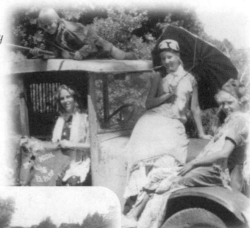

Of course, truck rides were a major part of his funeral day celebration (below).

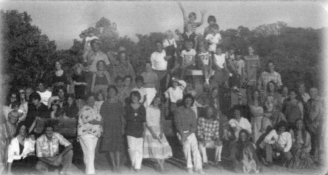

Grandchildren and friends dress up in vintage clothes for a truck ride.

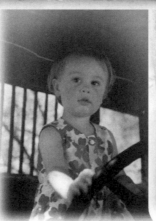

70 years later the truck is still running! New generations, including great-granddaughter, Mia and friends, Rose and Apaulo, dream of being at the helm of Pappy's old truck—a legacy of good times from another era.

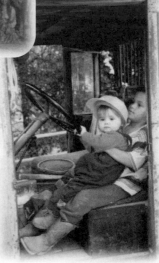

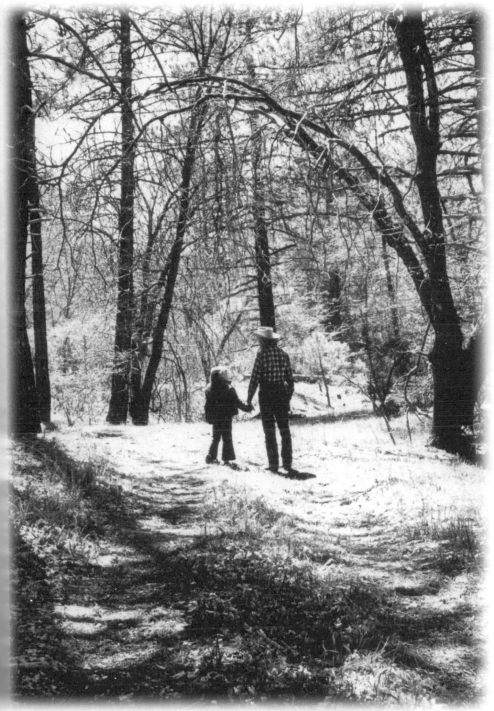

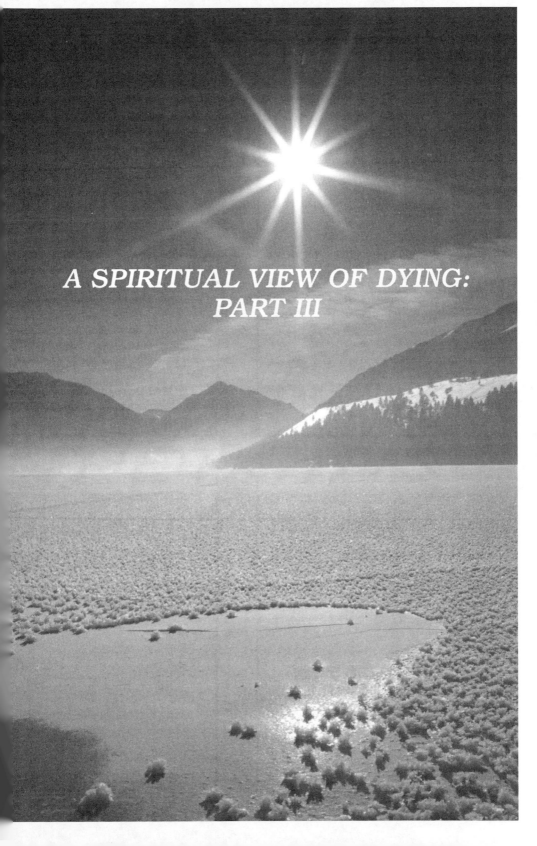

A SPIRITUAL VIEW OF DYING:
PART III

PREPARING FOR THE JOURNEY

The last years of our lives we are loosening up. Our spirit is moving beyond the body and preparing for our birth back to the other side as surely as the mother's body softens and opens as the birth time draws near. The elders can seem to lose their focus for earthly matters. Indeed, the sharpness of holding one's attention narrowly drawn to the minutiae of daily life fades as one prepares to step back to take in the larger picture. It is a natural process. The elder is preparing for a gaze that can encompass the soulscape, that can go across the threshold and begin to take in loved ones on the other side and cross over into the future.

As their inner world widens toward the spiritual world, myths and fairy tales can be of great support to the elderly and dying, if they are open to hearing them. Myths, stories and fairy tales have been distilled from oral tradition, from a long ago time when human beings had a more innate sense of the soul and spiritual world than we do today. Our modern self-centered intellectuality can limit our spiritual perceptions, unless we use it wisely to direct our awareness consciously toward a higher awareness.

*A fairy tale is about the human soul—**one** human soul. The characters in it represent all the aspects of our individual soul, the great classic struggles we have to let our highest and holiest (Prince, princess, king, queen, good fairy, etc.) shine into our basest and cruelest nature (giant, witch, monster, dragon) and to master them with courage and goodness. The tales are picture stories of our journey of life, our Quest and our trials to find if we have the perseverance, honesty and faith to triumph over despair and weakness. This is why young children thrive on such stories, for the archetypal pictures have a resonance of the soul and spirit world they have just come from. (Here I am not speaking of altered Disney versions of the tales. Children need to form their **own** images inwardly. They should only be given those fairy tales that they can enjoy in a good way and which are appropriate for their age). One lady was blessed as a little child with many fairy tales told to her by her grandmother. At eighty she told me, "Fairy tales are the rock of my old age!" She recognized how vital an inner life she had compared to her more impoverished contemporaries without such a heritage. The transformative pictures that nourished her in childhood enlivened her elder years with their rich inner relevance.*

As we age and near the threshold, not unlike the young child, we can move back into picture consciousness and become sensitive to images resonating out of the soul world. Universal soul stories are the source and power of true myth and fairy tale. Such stories can give nourishment and support long after the individual can no longer draw pleasure from abstract intellectual or scientific concepts that may have occupied their lives. A dear friend of mine, a priest, once read fairy tales to a slowly dying world-renowned physicist as he lay in the twilight between this world and the next. This may well have given the scientist more support than several worldly honors.

While I do not recommend reading a fairy tale to anyone, young or old, if the reader cannot feel some resonance with the story, (we are often put off by violence and the lack of logical earthly sense), it is worth trying to find one that does feel right.* It can be uplifting for many elders to receive such stories from someone who cares rather than the hours of endless, mindless television they are subjected to in so many cases.

When people come near to dying, they will often speak out of this inner world of symbolic pictures, and may give images to convey their impending transition. It is the language of metaphor. One man told his daughter, "I'm going to the pigeon fair, but I've only got one ticket." Another spoke of "looking for the spring flowers, or we must go to the park." A young athlete wrote on the margins of the TV sports guide, "out of the game by Sunday" (when he died). Others may speak with metaphors from work or hobbies such as taking the boat, or catching the plane. But by far the most universal sentiment expressed is about "going home," in reality going back to their spiritual home.

The miraculous embodiment of the spirit in a human being is an amazing process. We can watch its development in the growing capacities of the young child, then through the gradual fruition of a lifetime of experience, which, hopefully, ripens into wisdom and blessing for others. In the final years, there is often the gradual preparation for the journey back to another existence. If we have a sense for this spiritual journey, we can have more patience with the process of the loved ones who are leaving earthly life.

145

When we can age in wisdom, the expansion of spirit beyond the body can bring an equanimity, a patience, an ability to live beyond narrow self-interest and move into caring for humanity at large. There can be a mellowing of old intensities with more tolerance, more acceptance of others with all their weaknesses, and a growing tender appreciation of every human journey. Our elders may not all retain their ability to calculate, or to follow technical abstractions as they once did in the middle of life. But if they have retained wonder and devotion for life and, like the old Chinese proverb, "keep a green bough in their heart so the singing bird can come," then they can bless us all in old age. Surely the world needs more of such blessing.

Special stories could include the Grimm's stories of The Frog Prince, Star Money, Mother Holle, The Star Dollar, The Tailor in Heaven, Ash Girl, Snow White, Beauty and the Beast, Grandfather Death, Iron Hans, and Hansel and Gretel, stories by Clairssa Pincola Estes, The Radiant Coat and Other Tales, and Skeleton Woman, (from Women Who Run With the Wolves), The Three Candles of Little Veronica, by Manfred Kyber, The Day The Sun Rose, Leaf, by Nigel, by Tolkien, In The Ever After, Fairy Tales and the Second Half of Life. by Alan B. Chinan, as well as other native American legends, stories and folk tales which have pictures of death and transformation as the theme.

GETTING THE STORY

One of the greatest gifts we can give our elders and the dying is to be there for their "story." In loosening and preparing to leave their body, older people move onto a plateau not unlike the place where the incarnating child is coming in. This time of life seems to stir deep layers of the memory and can bring up to the surface buried childhood events with great clarity. While the elderly often cannot remember yesterday, the past can stand out vividly in their inner pictures. It is a precious window of opportunity to gather long ago stories of their lives.

Regardless of the age of the dying person, as they approach the threshold, there is a deep unspoken longing to round off the life, to make whole, to review and to make closure. In the summing up, along with the sense of achievement and accomplishment, there are almost always regrets, sorrows, and disappointments around unresolved issues and relationships, and a longing to have done more. It is a blessing to have someone who can listen and bear witness to the process. Certainly the listener is not called upon to judge, dismiss lightly, negate or suppress the process, or even to empathize to excess, but simply to be there and bear witness. The difficult issues need to surface too, like dark snags, branches of old trees rising to the surface from craggy logs deep in the river of the unconscious. Let them rise up and flow and release on the eddies of conversation, leaving a clear space for the dying.

Of course, it is certainly true that the listener can often get caught in the "double" nature of the elder or the dying one with his or her repetitive obsessions and complaints, but a good listener can help move things along with a good question; "How old were you when that happened?, How did you feel about that?, What did the others do then? Can you describe the place? What did you do after that? or statements like, "You were really needed then," and so forth.

The chance to be heard for this summary life review is truly a blessing and the one who is there to listen and participate is deeply benefited as well. It can be a rare and precious time for both parties involved. One of the most deeply human acts we can share is to bear such witness to another's biography.

Even when the elder moves into dementia, you can still stay with them. Frankly, I think it a Godsend when the paralyzed and bedridden can move in their *minds to another place, even if it is wandering from the harsh reality of their situation. Their wanderings can also be efforts to escape the cold, technological sounds and sterility of medical settings they may have to endure while others are caring for them.*

Listening, touching, being there and bearing witness to the journey, these are major gifts we can give to those culminating their lives, for these gestures are all unique and wonderful powers of being human. The elders and other friends who are in the process of dying give us great opportunities to develop ourselves with love and ever deeper humanity.

THE THREE DAYS AFTER DEATH—THE PROCESS

What is so unusual about the three days after death? Spiritually, many things are occurring for the one who has died. They are transitioning into a new state of existence through many experiences. As the vitality streams out of the body, it takes about three to three-and-a-half days time to dissolve into the general life essence of the world and universe.

The phenomenon occurs as follows. At death, the physical body is left behind and soon follows laws of the physical and mineral matter, namely rigidifying, breaking apart and decomposing. While we are alive, we are interpenetrated with a body of life, sometimes called the etheric body, through which we grow, metabolize, reproduce, unfold our physical form, derive formative vitality for our thinking, and reveal the patterns and possibilities of our life in time. Into this malleable and creative life body, which interpenetrates our physical organism, we impress our life experiences. It is a very creative and receptive memory aspect of our existence. When we die, the emerging of this life body from our physical body and its dissolving allows the tableau of our life experiences to surround and inform us. This phenomena can also be experienced by people who come near to death in an accident or a shock after which they often report, "I saw my whole life flash before my eyes." In these cases, however, the shock has rendered the etheric body only partly outside the physical so the tableau can only be fleetingly experienced.

When someone handles a dead body for the first time, it is surprising to find how incredibly heavy it feels, especially the head. Though the weight is the same as before death, the corpse is not animated by the body of life and therefore has become literally "dead" weight. One can then have the direct experience of how this compares with a body that has life. One can sense what a vitalizing aspect of our organism the life body is and how it gives us levity and vibrancy. All plants and animals have a life body, as well as humans.

The one who has died goes through two processes to begin with at death. First, the physical body is left behind by the emerging life body, soul and spirit. Secondly, after the three to three-and-one-half days, the life body, with the exception of a condensed extract that keeps a thread to our spiritual biography, dissolves away into the general life vitality of the planet.

Now soul and spirit move into a new phase where the spirit will review the results of the lifetime over a much longer period. This level of soul "schooling" entails experiencing the feelings of those we impacted in life; that is, what it was like for others to experience us, our effect on others in all aspects, both positive and negative. This realization and broader awareness lead the soul to a higher consciousness and insight into the life just lived, and the desire to make resolves for the future. Along with this self knowledge, there is a necessary purging or catharsis of the addictions and strong desires which drove the soul through the earthly senses, but which are no longer valid in a spiritual existence, indeed are hindrances to moving further into spiritual realms. Thus, the birth into pure spirit has many stages.

The sacredness of the three days after death is recognized in many diverse ancient cultures and religions. While in Jewish tradition burial occurs the day after death, there is also a special ceremony (tahara) where a devout group of caregivers wash and prepare the body. Obviously, in warm countries it may also be the custom to bury sooner. Yet there is an etheric process occurring during this time. I have had the experience, more than once, especially working with bodies that have not been embalmed and therefore have not had the features set through preservatives, of seeing some astounding changes during the three days. Not infrequently elders of eighty or ninety years look as young as thirty-five on the second and third day. Faces can sometimes move into expressions of incredible wisdom and peace (or not). When the process is complete (and it is usually quicker in small children), it is very obvious that it is complete and it is clearly time for cremation or burial.

If we are aware of this supersensible process in the three days after death, we can bring more consciousness during this time for those who have died, and bring respect for the absorbing and important task of the initial life review they are engaged in. One can sense it would be important not to try to plead with the deceased at this time for his or her energy, or to pull on them for support during this time in a direct way. If one has a world view that includes a guardian angel for everyone, then prayers and love can be sent through the angels during this time, insuring that the love and warmth will reach and support the one who has died, as well as reciprocate to the survivors, in all good ways. Of course, there is shock and grief, especially in sudden death, that the bereft survivors are experi-

encing. But if they can break free to accompany the loved one in the spirit with gratitude and hope, even if only for moments, it is a great gift for the one who has died.

It is also comforting to know that the life vitality which the loved one has offered up to universal life can aid in quickening the spiritual awareness and enhancing the consciousness of those left here in the world.

SPECIAL SIGNS IN NATURE

Some of the most special experiences that can happen around a death are unusual events that occur in nature. These can often be noted especially when the one who has died is an individual who has attended to his or her spiritual growth development and has given love in life. The vitality of the dying can sometimes be sensed in a response from the natural world.

In the three days following death, the life forces of the one who dies expand and dissolve into universal life, while the soul and spirit expand into a new existence as well. This can be a powerful, vital movement of energy from the physical to the spiritual plane, and one can look for reflections in nature. Our awareness of nature phenomena can be enhanced during this time as our sensitivities can be heightened by being so close to the threshold through the loved one's death.

Birds have always been the traditional messengers of the spiritual world. Flying free in heavenly space and back to earth is a picture of their interweaving gesture between this world and the next. In the fairy tale, it is the white dove that leads Snow White through the dark wood. It is the white dove that brings the olive branch to Noah; that descends upon Jesus at the baptism as a sign of the indwelling Christ, accompanied by the voice of God.

It is heart warming to be able to tell people to look for nature signs when a loved one crosses. They are often given a gift. Birds can come uncommonly close or butterflies appear. In Grandma Mary Edna's case a rainbow touched down in the back yard. The northwestern Native Americans have rich lore regarding the appearance of birds at various nodal points in life. They speak of the owl as the bird who calls the spirit back from this world to the next. Often with great historical figures, birds appear at death. When Joan of Arc died, a flock of doves assembled over the burning stake immediately afterward. When Rudolf Steiner, a great humanitarian of the 20th century, made his transition, flocks of doves appeared at his funeral. In 1226, as St. Francis lay unclothed upon the ground, bidding his weeping friars to gird him with a hair shirt and spread ashes over him, he died singing in a gentle voice, "Free my soul from prison, so that I may praise Thy name," and at the instant of his death a flock of skylarks arose above him and flew into the sky.

A touching occurrence happened for a friend of my mother's. The friend had a child late in life that was born at home and died within a few hours. My mother helped her through it all and ,soon afterward, the couple moved away.

When my mother died unexpectedly a few months later, I could not find the woman's address to notify her. It took me two months to locate it and to send her Lola's biography and news that she had died. She was stunned at the news, but as she was reading about Lola's life she looked out on the field and saw a bird lying there. She went to investigate and found a beautiful flicker, a type of large wood-pecker, that had died without a mark on it. She decided to take it to a nearby Native American museum. She gave it to the curator and then wandered through the museum. She was drawn to a life-sized carved wooden statue of a Native American healer, that was covered with flicker feathers. Across the base of the statue was carved the words "Spiritual Helper." She knew the message was from Lola. The timing could not have been more clear. Rudolf Steiner writes that, when the elderly die they keep us close with them as they go into the spiritual world and we remain in their care. The woman was deeply reassured that Lola would always be caring for her.

It is a surprise and delight to find how common these experiences are and everywhere you can find such stories if the question is asked. A woman told me that when her vital, red headed, gregarious father was dying, they could talk of love and memories, but not directly about spiritual things. She hoped she had been able to share the most supportive thoughts with him in their precious last days together. The day after he died, she walked in the redwoods and saw something she had never seen before—a flock of wild parrots, birds with a vigorous colorful style, just like her father. She knew all was well. When another friend's spunky mother died, a red cardinal kept coming to the window. An elderly lady had longed to travel abroad to the world center for the spiritual work she and her husband had shared in life. They had hoped to go there together, but he died first so she went alone. As she sat on a wall in front of the building thinking of him, a little bird came and sat upon her shoe and looked at her intently. She immediately felt the spirit presence and caring of her husband.

Dr. Viktor Frankl, the famous psychiatrist who survived the Nazi concentration camps and wrote the remarkable book, <u>Man's Search For Meaning,</u> related he had *no way of knowing if his wife was alive while he was in the camp. He writes,*

> "We were at work in a trench . . . for hours, I stood hack-
> ing at the icy ground. The guard passed by, insulting me. Once
> again, I communed with my beloved. More and more, I felt that
> she was present, that she was me. I had the feeling that I was
> able to touch her, able to stretch out a hand and grasp hers. The
> feeling was very strong that she was there. Then, at that very
> moment, a bird flew down silently and perched just in front of
> me, on the heap of soil which I had dug up from the ditch, and
> looked steadily at me."

My friend, Terry, whose four-year-old daughter, Emily, died of leukemia, receives her signs in butterflies, for it was a story of the butterfly that was the last story Emily heard from her mother before they took the child off life support. The butterflies are so omnipresent that we are no longer even surprised when we are talking together about Emily in the middle of winter, and Terry, who lives in New Jersey, sees a butterfly go by her window during our conversation! Or if I look out my window in California as we are speaking, a butterfly is there and often out of season as well. At a special gathering at Easter with many of us who had loved ones on the other side, a bird came at the evening meal and positively hammered on the window—after dark too!

It is affirming to ask about unusual experiences that coincide with a death and find that many people have had some very special incidents happen. May all these thoughts give an awareness of the many ways Mother Nature can give signs to bring comfort and hope in our grieving for our loved ones.

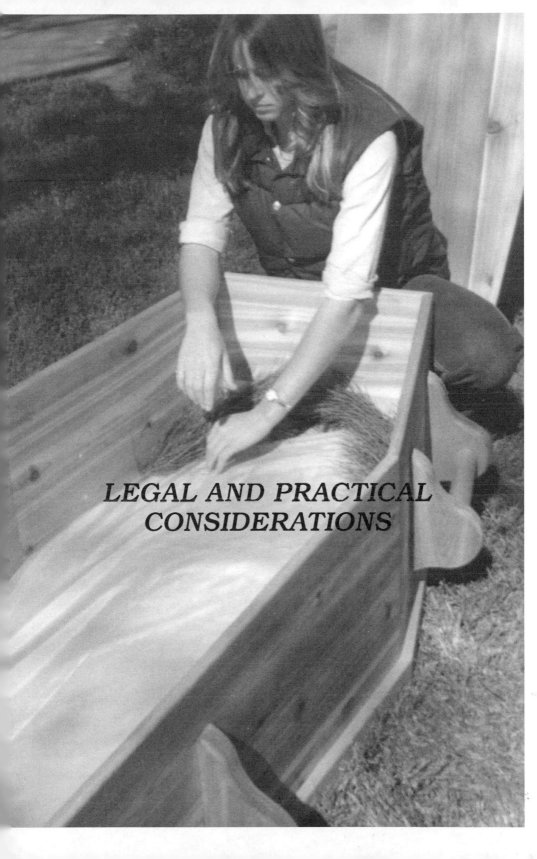

*LEGAL AND PRACTICAL
CONSIDERATIONS*

Building a Casket

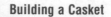

It is very fulfilling to make a casket for loved ones and friends in the community. Not only is it a real gift of practical caring, but provides a beautiful handmade casket for much less than one could be purchased. There are many types of casket solutions, from simple cardboard ones to elaborate metal containers. The two models shown here were created by our sons and can be built by skilled craftspersons.

However, a simple box can suffice. It needs to be at least 62 feet long, 24–29 inches wide, and a minimum of 14-inches high. I prefer 15-inch height so the person's face has ample room in a casket with a flat lid. For quickly made handles, holes can be drilled in the sides and a sturdy rope run through and knotted tightly inside, leaving enough slack in the rope to get a good grip to carry the casket. In building any casket it is important to use screws instead of nails in all four corners, top and bottom, for extra sturdiness. The same applies for attaching wooden handles. Screws can be countersunk and the holes carefully filled with matching wood filler.

Gary makes Pappy's casket

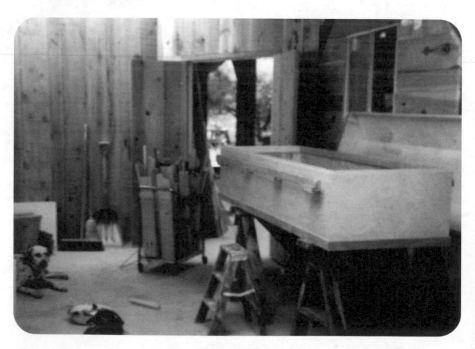

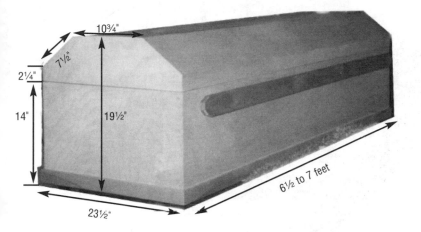

This casket requires two sheets of 3/4 inch plywood. Plywood comes in a variety of veneers, birch, oak, etc. These dimensions are for a small to medium-sized person so consider the requirements. The mitered edges on the lid can be cut on a table saw. In this model the box is built first and then the lid cut off afterward. Glue and nails are used except as noted on corners and handles where sheetrock screws are used. If a solid wood trim strip is added on the inside edge to help hold the lid in place, it needs to be angled slightly in so the lid can go on and off easily.

These dimensions are minimal, the wider the better up to 29 inches wide but the doorways to be maneuvered through will be a determining factor. (Remember caskets can't go around corners without a lot of room to turn. In this design, solid wood handles can be sculpted and need a full inch distance from the casket to allow for a good hand hold when carrying.

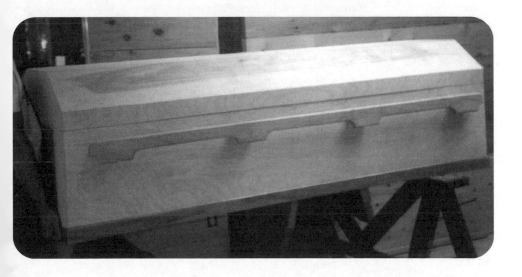

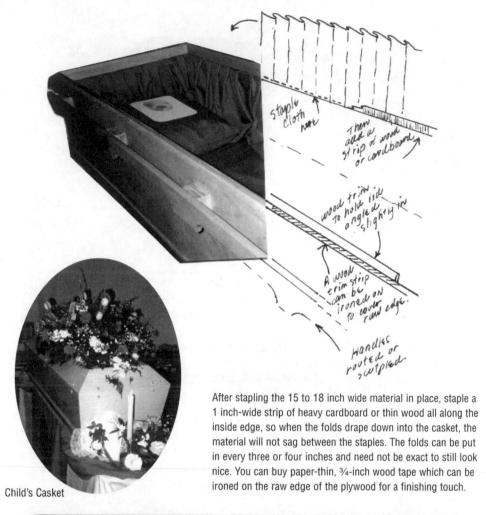

staple cloth here

Then add a strip of wood or cardboard

wood trim to hold lid angled slightly in

A wood trim strip can be ironed on to cover raw edge.

Handles routed or sculpted.

Child's Casket

After stapling the 15 to 18 inch wide material in place, staple a 1 inch-wide strip of heavy cardboard or thin wood all along the inside edge, so when the folds drape down into the casket, the material will not sag between the staples. The folds can be put in every three or four inches and need not be exact to still look nice. You can buy paper-thin, ¾-inch wood tape which can be ironed on the raw edge of the plywood for a finishing touch.

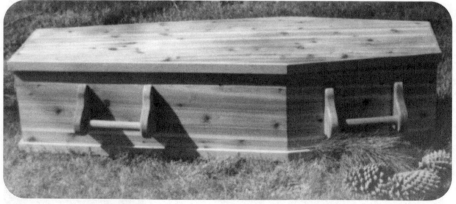

This casket design begins with 14 or 15 inch squares on each end. It tapers out to 26–28 inches at the widest point (at ⅓ of the casket length). Overall width, including handles should be no more than 29 inches.

LEGAL AND PRACTICAL CONSIDERATIONS

My threshold work began with the deep feelings I had as an artist that this final celebration of a human life should be as beautiful, and uplifting as it could possibly be for any given situation. This is what motivated and inspired me to become involved. There was a strong sense that the space where the body would be should have touches of beauty through flowers, pictures, and lovely color to help create a mood of quiet and peace for prayer, contemplation, and honoring the loved one with last good-byes. At the very least, I feel there should be simplicity and order in the place where the casket and vigil take place. Equally appropriate, I feel, is the natural flow of family life taking place nearby.

Home death, as home birth, is certainly not for everyone. Whatever arrangements take place, they need to be appropriate for that individual and the family that is involved. This is offered so people will know there are choices, some of which they might choose if they knew it is possible to do so. For some, these may be ways that they feel they could not possibly consider. Yet when the time comes, they may find the strength, from both inner and outer resources, to create the final ritual for their loved ones in a different way than they might have imagined they could.

For many years I have been asked to make this material available. I have hesitated to do so because I did not want to write anything about bodily care that could be shocking or dismaying to the survivors. My greatest concern was that a sense of dignity, rightness, and fulfillment of the life of the deceased be the focus of those participating in caring for their loved ones at death.

The world has become more explicit about the harsh realities of life and perhaps many people are better able to deal with the grosser aspects of physical experiences. I do ask, however, that the reader take these writings with especially sensitive caring for the survivors, how each aspect may affect them, and in which aspects it may be appropriate to involve them. Please take this information with reverence for each human spirit, for the dignity of life, and with openness to the reality of spirit in which they are offered.

Every Funeral is Unique

Every death is individual. The circumstances around the death and the ceremony afterward vary widely. Not only is the deceased involved, but there are also various constellations of families and friends, all with their views and opinions. Some have more responsibility than others for carrying out the funeral process. Ideally, there will be a consensus on procedure. Hopefully, the deceased's wishes are considered, although some people who have stated they didn't want a ceremony of honoring to take place when they died, may well find it a blessing in their new state of being when thoughtful and prayerful work is done on their behalf by those who are remembering them.

When an individual family member is hoping for some of the aspects that we outline here to be done, but is unable to make it work in his or her family network, I encourage the family member to quietly carry a spiritual view as he or she goes into the situation. Even without words a person can maintain a prayerful connection to the deceased loved one, and try to give support to those who are having a struggle with the death. It is helpful if there can be three days before cremation or burial. This will usually seem like a reasonable request to make.

What is shared here is a community process which has been deeply appreciated by many families. This work has enriched community life immeasurably, and those involved have strongly felt it has been spiritually beneficial to the one who has died. Death is like birth. We hope for it to be as ideal as possible, but there is no perfect situation. We all do the best we can in any circumstance. We offer these possibilities for choice, and for consideration of whatever aspect of this process may be appropriate for your unique family situation.

Know Your State Laws

Laws regarding caring for your loved ones and friends at death vary from state to state, some existing to benefit the huge and powerful funeral industry. I usually try to deal with small, independent funeral homes that are open to personal requests and service. However, they are increasingly being bought up by large corporations.

Ideally, if you are planning a home death, you will have worked out the necessary procedure well before the death. There will need to be arrangements with the doctor and hospice. You will need to know where to go for the death certificate, what county offices to go to for permits, and so forth. Hopefully, there can also be a supportive friend who knows what to do. It is imperative to be working with a physician, if you wish to die at home, because nearly all states require autopsies if you die at home and are not in touch with your physician a few weeks before death. Under hospice care this requirement is fulfilled. The doctor must state the cause of death on the certificate. Without the medical authority to sign for the reason for dying, criminal causes may be assumed by authorities and an autopsy required. Avoid an autopsy if at all possible. Not only is it invasive, but you will be tied to the coroner's timetable to get the body back if you wish to have it at home. Autopsies are almost always required in accidental death, but we have had some success where the cause was obvious and we have asked for an exception on religious grounds.

Through joining a local memorial society you can stay informed about funeral costs and services in your area. There is a national hot line where a state watch regarding all funeral issues is maintained with up to date information. I recommend calling as you make your preparations because laws vary from state to state. The hotline number is Funeral Consumers Alliance (FAMSA) 1-800-765-0107. The website at www.funeral.com

Remember the purpose of funeral professionals is to take pressure off the families at this intense time in life. They take care of the issues around transportation, paper work, etc. and many of them do it very well. To do the things we are speaking of here truly requires a group of friends who can make it beautiful and honoring without adding extra stress to the family situation. Sometimes with a small funeral home or crematory service, it is possible to employ them on a limited basis to fill out and file the death certificate, or to transport the body, or remove it if stairs are involved, for example.

The following are some threshold groups and businesses that give support for a home death and vigil.

In Silver Springs, Maryland, Crossings (301) 593-545, deathcrossings@msn.com or website at www.crossings.net.

In Sebastopol, California, Final Passages (707) 824-0268, finalpassages@softcom.net or website at www.finalpassages.org. (They sell *Handbook for Creating A Home Funeral* and casket plans.)

In Sacramento, California, The Threshold Circle, Heidi Boucher (916) 967-7095, heidiboucher@aol.com

In Boulder, Colorado. Natural Transitions Funeral Guidance (303) 245-4886.

In Minneapolis, Minn., Twin Cities Threshold Group (651) 633-0432 Dennis & Marianne Dietzcl, dld@visi.com; Linda Bergh, lindabergh@aol.com.

Getting The Body Released

Even though many states allow families to care for their own dead, and have legal statutes that give the right for the disposition of the body to the next of kin, you may still encounter difficulty in getting a hospital or nursing home to release the body directly to the family. Most institutions will tell you they will only release it to a funeral home operator.

If you plan to bring your loved one home at death after a stay in a hospital or nursing home, go over the process with the institution involved *prior* to the death if it is at all possible. State that you have the right under the law to claim the body (you can find the exact statute for your state from FAMSA) and that you wish to do so for mourning and religious reasons. Make this known to the patient advocates. Ask exactly how this can take place in that institution down to all the details such as how the removal can take place, the necessary paper work to do and so forth. Talk it through.

If they still refuse to acknowledge your rights, it may be necessary to have a letter from an attorney citing your rights under the law. Take numerous copies of such a letter and distribute to all levels of personnel at the institution. Hospitals and nursing homes do not want law suits, but it may take this step to get them to comply. Of course, you can always resort to a funeral home removal if you have to, and hopefully there will only be a minimum charge for the service. You may be able to get the funeral home to come to the institution and do the mediating paperwork, so you can take the body directly. Lisa Carlson of FAMSA (1-800-765-0107) is a capable and experienced advocate who will call authorities on behalf of families whose rights are not being acknowledged.

The Paper Work

It is imperative, if you wish to do death care for family and friends, to have all the legal paper work in order. The most crucial item is the death certificate. Usually these are readily available to funeral homes and the doctor, although in some cases you can obtain them from the county. However, individuals may face difficulties in trying to do so. In our state, California, one can sometimes pick up a practice one at county health departments and have the data ready. Then when the event occurs you transfer the data to the death certificate that the doctor signs. Ideally, the doctor could have the certificate for you to fill out ahead of time. Then when the death occurs he or she could simply sign and state the cause of death and you would be ready to go for filing, The doctor is required to sign it within fifteen hours in

California. However, we have often encountered problems with the doctor not having a death certificate and have faced the necessity to run back and forth between their office and the county to complete the work.

Taking care of the paper work is a service the funeral home provides. If you are filling it out yourself, you need to know it must be filled out in ink or typed with NO ERRORS OR CORRECTIONS. Also the writing cannot touch the lines around each space as the data will likely be computerized later.

You will need to supply the full name of the deceased, birth date and place of birth, full names of the parents and where they were born. There is a space for the occupation for the deceased and where the ashes will be located. Once you have this document, go to the county health department offices or the bureau of Vital Statistics, file the form and get permits for cremation or burial and for transportation as required in that state. Requirements for each state can be obtained by calling the FAMSA hotline I-800-765-0107 or www.funerals.org/famsa. Get started on death certificate data and process early, as it can take even days to get all the signatures and information finished and filed.

When Death Occurs

The time just following the death is emotional and holy. A spiritual birth has just occurred. It is not a time for frantic preparations as these are not needed by the one who has died. It is most helpful if the survivors can simply try to be open to what has just taken place spiritually. You do not have to call the undertaker to come immediately, though the doctor who will sign the death certificate must be notified as soon as reasonably possible. The only things to do immediately are to close the eyes (if needed) and close the mouth. For this purpose a towel can be rolled up and placed under the chin to prop it closed. Keep the head tilted on a pillow and this will also help to keep the mouth closed. Often a kerchief can be used to tie up the chin with a knot on top of the head, but sometimes this sets the mouth uncharacteristically. However, it is a measure that may be needed. Fold the arms over the mid-section and the hands over one another. One can then take time for prayer and quiet until it is time for bathing and dressing. If there is a need for cleanup from the bowels, bathing would take place sooner.

Buying or Making the Casket

Do not be talked into an elaborate casket if that is not what is needed. Many funeral directors will not show the lesser priced ones unless you request to see them. Ask to be left alone in the casket showroom to make your selection. There are many ways to make a plain casket beautiful. Most plain caskets are press board covered with gray and these usually work out well. Lovely silk cloths or other cloth may be used to give a richness to a casket and the table or bed it is resting on. The table or bed can be draped and there are always flowers to go on the top of the casket. Caskets can be purchased from mortuaries, funeral supply stores and on the Internet(www.undertakers). You can expect to get some pressure to purchase a casket from the mortuary you are working with. Find out if the funeral home will make a surcharge to you if you are providing your own casket rather than buying one of theirs. There are also various types of heavy cardboard containers available, if transportation to the crematorium is all that is needed. These can also serve for "lying in honor" during the three days at home and can provide family members with an opportunity to paint or decorate the casket themselves. Simple pine caskets are available for purchase too.

We have made beautiful wooden caskets in our community, some by groups working all night on short notice. But it may prove easier to buy one, depending on the circumstances. In some states where re-use of caskets is allowed, people use no casket at all, and after the vigil the body is lifted into a casket for transport

Considering the Room

One of the first interesting things that comes up with home death is getting the casket in and out of the house. One can always tip the casket sideways bringing it into the room, but that is not what you want to do when carrying it out with the body. Often there are hallways and corners you can't go around. Many a body has ended up in the living or dining area because the casket would not go in the back bedroom. If there seems to be a problem in having the casket in the main living area, a screen can be found to provide more privacy for visitors. One needs to also plan how the casket will be taken from the house. If there are good-sized windows available in the bedroom, these can provide an option for taking the coffin out. If getting out the front door is a problem, there may be a need to go out the back yard to the street to load it in a van. Most caskets, including handles, are just the width of a normal doorway. Anyone making a casket should consider this, as well as not making it too large to fit in the door of the furnace at the crematorium.

Preparing the Casket

If the casket is home made it should be prepared with some padding in the bottom. Commercial varieties use excelsior, fine wooden shavings. I usually find an old wool blanket or mattress pad for the initial padding as there can be moisture from the body and an absorbent material is desirable. Cedar shavings might be used in the bottom of the casket too, providing a pleasant scent. The sheet used to transfer the body into the casket will go on top of whatever material is in the bottom. It can be tucked in at the sides and is hardly visible. A medium-sized pillow is necessary as it is very awkward and inartistic to have the body completely flat. A cover may be made for the pillow that is a pleasing color or styles for that individual. Otherwise, white is always appropriate. Be sure, of course, that the person's nose and head will not be too high when the lid is closed. Though not necessary, we have often put sweet smelling branches in the casket. Rosemary is ideal for this, as well as fragrant cedar, pine, juniper or eucalyptus.

When making your own casket, you can staple cloth to the inside. Tucks may be folded in as it is stapled, which gives a pleasing effect in the drapery and give room for the dry ice underneath. Along the inside rim of the casket, staple the edge of the cloth in tucks three to four inches apart, and then let the cloth fall back down inside and over the staples so they are not visible. It helps to also staple a one to two inch strip of thin wood or heavy cardboard over the staples so the cloth stays flush with the edge and does not sag unevenly (See diagram). Most fabric is 36 inches wide and half of this (an 18 inch width) is just right for the drapery around the inside of the casket. For the bottom padding, the pillow and the drapery around the edges, I usually buy nine yards of fabric. Dry ice is put underneath the folds and wilted flowers can be tucked there as well.

About Rigor Mortis

Just as labor is a rhythmic process increasing in intensity to the time of birth, so dying is a rhythmic process reflecting the great ebbs and flows of blending back into universal existence. The spirit labors and breathes itself out of a body that is being shed. Earthly laws then prevail for the physical body as it goes from the living to the lifeless state and will shortly begin to disintegrate. Conversely, the vitality and spirit of the individual are now under universal spiritual laws. Rigor mortis conditions will vary widely with different people. Generally within an hour or two after the death, rigor mortis will begin to set in. This is why we try to close the eyes and set the mouth in place in a natural way soon after death. There will be a first hardening of the body after a few hours, and twenty four hours or so later there will be a relaxing again and then a rhythmic re-hardening. Sometimes we need to attend to the mouth which may tend to open on the second day. If necessary a few drops of super glue (which bonds to skin) can be used to help keep it closed. Funeral homes use a small plastic mouth former that can help keep it closed too, as well as little plastic caps to help keep the eye lids closed. These may be available to you. However, they are not always necessary.

Washing and Preparing the Body

The bodies most easily preserved without embalming are those that are thin and dehydrated. This can often naturally be the case when the dying person has taken little food or water in the last days. This is a natural response in dying as the organ systems are shutting down, and, near death, the swallowing reflex no longer functions. Those bodies which are corpulent, or where there is extensive cancer or open sores, will tend to deteriorate more quickly. That is not reason not to have them home for the three days. It just requires extra awareness in preparation of the body, covering the sores well, keeping the casket cool, and perhaps closing the casket sooner.

The body can be washed with warm water using only a little soap and cotton swabs where extra cleaning is needed. It takes two people to handle the body easily. Moving the body over is done just as it is done with any bedridden patient, by pulling up and bending one leg (which will be on top when they are rolled) and rolling them onto their side. Expect to use a number of towels and wash rags, especially if the hair needs washing. Obviously, plastic bags can be placed around to keep from soaking the bed. In some religious views, it is important to use special oils for anointing, preparing and wrapping of the body. If there are open sores (e.g. bedsores) these need to be treated with some kind of drying powder (not too strong in smell) and covered with gauze and plastic wrapping and then covered well with tape. There is an excellent wound dressing, which forms a clear second skin over wounds and can be used to cover the wound. I usually find on dry skin that duct tape works well for a final taping over. This is assuming this area will be covered with clothing. Use covering of some sort over these places, or if there are skinned places on a hand, simply place the other hand over it.

Sometimes, especially after a long labor of dying, there can be some drainage of blood and mucous from the mouth, usually less than a cup. This discharge will usually occur naturally when the body is rolled over for cleaning. The mouth can be swabbed a bit and then closed well. There can also be some leakage of bowel fluids from the anus. With a rubber glove, take a large amount of cotton (an amount about the size of a soft ball or grapefruit) and pack it carefully into the anus. This will prevent any problem, especially when the body is moved. If the person has been bedridden, there are usually disposable diapers available. I usually put one of those on too as an added protection. It is always a question whether to put an elder's false teeth back in. On the second or third day after death, the mouth will be somewhat concave if it is not done; on the other hand it may seem just as natural without the teeth. If there is a moustache it would hardly be noticeable. This should be done at the time of bathing.

Close loved ones will have a sense of what will be the appropriate clothing to dress the body. With two people, the dressing can be easily managed. Belts are not necessary, nor more than minimal undergarments. If a person is very large or a dress or suit is tight or difficult to get on, the clothing can be partially slit down the back and tucked in around the body and it will look fine.

Placing The Body in the Casket

If using a home made casket which does not have a split lid (so only the top half of the body is shown), then cover the bottom half of the body with a shawl, a blanket or artistic covering of some sort as the legs and feet detract from the emphasis on hands and face. The hands can be folded across one another in a natural way across the abdomen.

Ideally, four people can lift the body into the casket, obviously depending on the weight of the person, two on each side. In a pinch, three can do it. A strong man or woman with a long reach can hold the head and the weight of the torso while two others, one on either side, can assist the lift. A sturdy, dry sheet or blanket should be placed under the body after bathing. This is then rolled up close to each side of the body. The rolled cloth gives a good grip for those who are lifting the body. This sheet or blanket can be left in the casket under the body, as it is awkward to remove it.

Using Dry Ice for Preservation

If there is to be a three day vigil, it is good to have dry ice to help cool the casket and the environment for the body. The body can be kept at home for twenty-four hours or so without any measures being taken if the temperature and humidity in the room are not extreme. If the time is expected to be longer, then dry ice can be used. Given the processes that are happening for the spirit of the individual, we want to keep it as natural as possible, at the same time keeping down odors which could make it unpleasant for visitors and survivors. Sometimes people leave the individual on the bed and put dry ice in pillow slips underneath the body. However, it is easier to control the coolness of the environment around the body with a casket. Also the body without a casket has to be moved into a container after three days which can sometimes present problems. Blankets placed underneath to begin with can help to make the then transfer easier.

I prefer to try to keep the body from freezing as much as possible to work with the natural process, and therefore do not put the ice under the body which will freeze the lower half. The torso and abdomen are the main areas to keep cool and therefore slabs of ice are placed primarily around the upper body under the folds of the casket lining. I usually begin with thirty pounds of ice (available through super markets, or it can be found in the yellow pages). Dry ice can burn and must be handled with rubber or other protective gloves. If there is a large piece of ice that needs to be broken, a cleaver or hammer will work. The ice usually comes in slabs about a foot square and one to two inches thick. Wrap the ice well in three or four large pages of newspaper and then put it in a plastic bag. DO NOT CLOSE THE BAG. Leave the open end facing to one side. The ice evaporation needs to work to cool the environment. The plastic bag is only to prevent excess moisture from accumulating in the casket and makes the frosted packages easier to handle when replacing the ice.

When there are disposable bed pads available from the care of a bedridden patient, I usually place these between the wrapped ice and the side of the casket. This is because the ice can tend to form condensation on the outside of the casket from the intense cold and this padding gives extra insulation. Bubble pack used for protection in wrapping packages works very well for this purpose too. The slabs of ice can be packed all around the body and under the pillow beneath the head. The whole purpose is to keep the environment cool to slow deterioration. Obviously, it is better to have the body in a cool room and not by a heater vent or where sunshine is directly on it.

During the second day, the ice bags are removed and changed. This time usually twenty to twenty-five pounds works well and that may be all that will be needed for the whole process. As situations vary in many ways, someone needs to keep checking on the state of things at least once each day. (I usually do all the changing alone in the room or with a helper, as I try to keep it as artistic as possible for the family, though sometimes it is therapeutic for a family member to help.) At the end of the second day there may be swelling of the abdomen. Gases from anaerobic bacteria in the stomach and intestines can cause this. If there seems to be extreme need, I will sometimes place some wrapped ice directly on the stomach to inhibit the process and cover with a cloth or blanket, but I prefer not to unless it is really necessary. If odors become a problem the casket can be closed. If it is hard to maintain a cool temperature in the room, the casket can be closed when there are no visitors.

About Embalming

Most people have the impression embalming is required by law. In virtually all states it is not. There are, however, many states that have time limits (12–48 hours) that you can have the body at home without embalming or dry ice. Embalming is a rigorous and invasive procedure in which inner organs are perforated and all the bodily fluids are drained out and replaced with a fluorescent pink formaldehyde to give the impression of color in the skin. The strength of the formaldehyde can vary and no solution will permanently preserve the body. In some cases, embalming may seem the best and easiest solution for a funeral, especially with people coming from far away. It can be asked that the strength of the solutions used be minimal to get through the brief time period involved. It is helpful for the body not to be embalmed when this is a reasonable choice. Artificial preservation is not the natural separation process of the organism on all levels. However, just as all births are not the same, so every aspect of the family's needs and those of the deceased will be part of the consideration about this choice.

If You Choose Not to Embalm

If the choice is made not to embalm the body, yet the family still wants to have a vigil at the funeral home, you will probably find yourself facing certain attitudes from the morticians. They often will not want an unembalmed body to be viewed, except for identification or brief closure with the immediate family. They will usually provide a room in the mortuary for visitation, but they prefer to embalm the body if the casket is to be open. Usually they will only allow you to visit at certain hours. Most funeral businesses will not allow a vigil through the night because they do not want to deal with insurance issues or the extra cost of a night watchman. Therefore, if you want to have a round-the-clock vigil with an un-embalmed body (or an embalmed body for that matter), you have to do it yourself at home or in a church. This is one of the main reasons we began our own threshold work in our community.

The funeral home will, of course, deliver the body to the home if you wish and will perform all the services you request: dressing, casketing, transport,

169

etc. They will, however, charge you a substantial basic fee for their involvement. They are required by law to give the customer a complete break down of their charges, so you can choose those services you wish to pay for and what you might want to do yourself. We have had a number of home deaths with no professional involvement other than cremation. However, all the legal paper work must be done in order to do so.

If you wish to have the body at home for twenty-four hours or so following the death, and then take it to the funeral home, they have a cold room where the body can be kept for three days before cremation. It can be helpful to deal with a funeral home that has the cold room and crematorium in the same facility. When people are unable to have the body at home and do not plan a vigil, I often advise having the body kept in the cold room at the mortuary for the three days. They can then have a closed casket for the funeral, or it can then be transported to the crematorium or cemetery. In such a case, the family can do their remembrances and prayers for the deceased at home and have rituals of remembrance there or at a church.

Preparing the Room

When someone has died at home, it is a very natural impulse for the family to have a burst of energy to create a beautiful space in the wake of the departure. The challenge of taking whatever space is available and making it artistic and aesthetically pleasing has been one of the most interesting and fulfilling parts of my work. The casket is large and heavy and will take up room. It is awkward to have it placed on the floor. Sometimes the only thing big enough for it to rest on is a bed, or a futon or couch with strong wooden arms.

I always try to "listen" to what colors are the right ones for the person who has just passed and try to find a bedspread or sheets that seem harmonious. Sometimes, I buy material to drape beds or tables to make it beautiful. Obviously each family will have their own approach to this. I always try to remove or cover all electronic gadgets, computers, TV's, etc. These seem very out of place for this event. It is desirable to have tables at each end of the casket (or very tall candle holders) where candles can be placed to keep the body in light rather than in shadow. I have sometimes used end tables with a stack of large books to make it the right height and then covered the books and tables with cloth. Branches of pine or cedar can be used for decorating in the room as well.

Some Special Touches

It is hard to procure everything that may be needed at the last minute. This is why a Threshold Committee, or a friend who has a sense of the full scope of what needs to be done, is an invaluable support for a home death. Obviously, planning ahead can make these special days more peaceful and allow the survivors to concentrate on being there spiritually rather than dealing with the details of death certificate information, making choices about a casket, and so forth.

In each case, a family will simply do the best they can with what they have. However, it is both spiritually helpful and beautiful to include certain touches. Rosemary is a wonderful herb to have present in the room in bouquets and in the casket. Rosemary oil can also be placed in vases or bowls of water. The three-day process of the dissolution of the life forces is enhanced by the water nearby. Having the naturally fragranced water in the room is supportive to the process. Roses are always appropriate, reflecting the many layers of the soul and transmuted love. Pure rose water may be sprayed in the room. Carnations are bright cheerful flowers which stay fresh for a long time.

Beeswax candles are the most desirable if they can be found. Though expensive, the large candles can burn through the night, even up to 48 hours or more. It is good to have such natural light at either end of the casket, if this is feasible, so the body remains as much in light as possible. The family will often want to make a display of photos of the deceased to have nearby, along with mementos that had special meaning for them. It is a nice touch to leave a note for visitors with the full name of the one who has died and the birth and death dates.

I recommend that flowers placed in the casket be left in there, even though they wilt on the second or third day. They can be tucked under the folds of the casket drapery in that case. Not only have they been lovingly given by the one who placed them there, but they are giving up their life essence just as the one who has died and are supportive to the whole process.

The Vigil

The ideal we are striving for in a vigil is to create a continuous thread of conscious, spiritual, caring thoughts flowing to the one on the other side who is now finding his or her way into a new state of being. If a vigil is planned (it can be up to three days) it helps to have a friend take responsibility to set it up. The schedule, in hourly increments, should be kept near the phone in the home where the vigil takes place so people can call and make arrangements to come. Right after the death, the friend can make calls to those they feel would want to participate to get the initial schedule in place for the first hours. The first thing, however, is to inquire what hours the family may want and put them in the schedule, although they may not really know at that point.

It is best to have people read for a half-hour to an hour, and not more than two hours. It is fine if two readers come together and sit reading quietly. The hardest hours to fill are after midnight to dawn (hourly shifts are the most appropriate for this time). Readers with experience know how special keeping vigil at such hours can be. Hopefully, there will be some of these people in the community willing to take night hours. Those who read for the one who has died during these midnight to dawn hours make a significant contribution, for that is when the rest of the community is asleep. It is a special gift when someone is faithfully carrying this stream of thoughtful support through this time.

If someone cannot leave their home to come and read at night, they can volunteer to awaken at a certain hour and read for the person from their own home. On the third day it is often hard to find readers for the night. When my father died we were all needing our sleep on the third night, and called our children in Sweden to read for those hours. They were night hours here but daylight hours for them! If a round-the-clock vigil is not a realistic possibility, perhaps someone can call friends of the deceased across the country and ask that a common prayer, a sacred text or Bible reading (the St. John gospel is always helpful) be offered by them at a certain time, which will vary with the time zones and help keep a stream of support going.

In our community, we arrange a comfortable chair and small light for visitors to read through the night. A lyre for playing quiet music is lovely to have available. Have a comfortable shawl for visitors for extra warmth when the room is very cool. The Bible, books such as Rudolf Steiner's about life after death, poetry, fairy tales, or other readings of a spiritual nature, especially those passages that were meaningful to the loved one who has died, can be read. It is especially nice if a guest book can be made available so those coming can sign their names and give comments. This will be a record of visitors who came for the special vigil and will be very meaningful to the family afterward.

Those helping the family need to be especially sensitive to times for the family to be alone with the body. The family needs to be encouraged to make their needs known to anyone there. In addition a large, readable card can be placed by the guest book such as the following:

PLEASE BE AWARE THAT FAMILY MEMBERS MAY NEED TIME HERE ALONE. IF SO, PLEASE CONTINUE YOUR READING IN THE LIVING ROOM WHERE IT WILL BE NO LESS HELPFUL AND APPRECIATED. THANK YOU SO MUCH FOR BEING HERE NOW FOR ALL OF US.

The Family.

The front door is usually left unlocked. A night light is left on, and instructions about the location of the room are posted with the encouragement to be quiet for the family's sake.

When people come to read for the first time they are usually full of trepidation. Almost always, they come away amazed at the peacefulness and the spiritual uplift they have gained by this vital life experience around death. They also have the fulfillment of knowing they have supported a family when it is most needed.

Cremation or Burial

Most people have formed their own opinions about choices for dealing with the body after death. It is probably fortunate for the planet, in lieu of space, that many people today choose cremation. However, some people feel strongly they wish burial and such wishes should to be honored. Once the three-day process is over, cremation completes the transformation to render the physical body back to ashes. As stated before, it can be recommended for a suicide that the body be buried. Also in hot countries and in the Jewish tradition, the burial takes place on the second day.

In many cemeteries there is a requirement that the casket be placed in a concrete vault in the ground, because cemetery keepers want to maximize the available space by stacking several caskets in one plot. Also they do not wish to have the ground sink in later as the caskets deteriorate. This would form depressions that make it more difficult to mow the lawns. But a cement vault can inhibit a natural return to the earth and certainly makes it a much longer process.

Above all, avoid pressure from mortuary salesmen to choose a sealed casket with rubber gaskets and a key-cranked lock. When the body cannot receive air to dry out and decay in a natural manner, the results are appalling and quite contrary to how the family had hoped to preserve the body. There are a few cemeteries that do not use caskets, instead wrapping the bodies in cloth for a simple and straight forward return to the earth. The graves are also unmarked so the whole area is like a lovely park. The family can ask questions about what is available to them through cemeteries in their area. For many people it is important to have a place to go to in the time after the loved one's death, and a place in a cemetery fulfills that need. It is a place for the survivors of the loved one to come to for a sense of closeness. Any location where the ashes are buried can serve this purpose, too. Some people like to keep the ashes at home about a year before making a final disposition, and this can seem to be a natural rhythm, too. It is often necessary to have permission to scatter ashes in certain places. Find out the legalities for your state. Ashes are a natural substance, and there is wisdom in the ancient saying, "dust to dust."

Closing the Casket

If there is a need because of seasonal heat, or the state of the body, to keep more coolness in, the casket can be closed during the night or during the day, when there are no visitors. Otherwise, if all is well, it may remain open for the three days of the vigil. Ideally, candles in addition to a small lamp, can provide soft lighting. Obviously, for the night time hours. candles need to be safe when burning. Closing the casket on the third day is a very poignant time for the family. Since it is the last view of the body and has a deep finality to it. I try to involve the family members who wish to be there, especially if there is not an official religious ceremony at this time. Usually, I place a silk cloth, or sheer cloth over the face and then place many of the flowers that have been brought over the three days over the body. (Of course, many bouquets may also need to go to the church for the services if that is part of the ritual). Special mementos and children's drawings, poetry, etc. may seem right to place in the casket. Once the casket is closed another step in closure is completed.

Some people have the whole farewell funeral ceremony at home and this can be a lovely time for someone to play or sing music, offer special poems and remembrances as well as religious readings and blessings by a minister or rabbi. The funeral can also be in a church setting where there is more room for friends to attend. Bringing flowers and setting things up at church can also be a task for the friends who are helping in a home death. The family may also wish to accompany the body to the crematorium. This aspect can be difficult, but deeply meaningful as well. At the crematorium, the casket is usually burned with the body. To some having a beautiful handmade casket burned may seem difficult, but another view is that it is a final and fitting gift of love for this completion process.

Taking Care of Yourself

The tremendous life changing experiences undergone by the constellation of survivors of a death cannot be underestimated. It is inevitable that everyone will be changed by the experience of the death of a loved one. If we choose to be involved in threshold work, we need to know the importance of sensible care for ourselves and for the remaining family. With the death of someone close to us, we are open to his or her dying experience and can be taken part way across the threshold into spiritual space along with the dying person. This is a gift, for we can have enhanced spiritual awareness in that expanded state. On the other hand, we need to stay grounded and remain here in our bodies in a healthy way.

We must be especially sensitive to the needs of survivors as well as their sensibilities when we are aiding in a home death. Try to keep an awareness of whether they are getting food, some rest, some quiet, a walk or other exercise, a time in nature or the garden, and time to sit with the body, shower or bathe, or receive a rub for their shoulders or a massage. The same applies to caring for ourselves, although we may be required to work long hours to make the event go well.

Survivors are often in shock and grief, especially with a sudden death. They are often also exhausted from long hours by the deathbed. They then require someone with the ability to do what needs to be done without making a lot of requests of them, while at the same time being sensitive to their needs. Though I always offer them the opportunity, I do not involve family members in care of the body unless they express a desire to do so. However, if they want to take this role for their loved one, it can be a wonderful catharsis, a beginning of healing and wholesome closure for them.

When we have loved ones cross to the other side we can feel torn with grief and hollowed out around our heart and solar plexus. The solar plexus is especially where we feel the effects from those who have died. It is recommended that a salve of copper ointment be applied to this area of the body for some days after the death. (available from Uriel Pharmacy, 262-642-2858, or Raphael Pharmacy, 916-962-1099). This gives a layer of protection for healing and reclaiming our own organism which has been so intimately intertwined with the deceased and their life forces. It is especially important to give extra support this way and also with images of protection around the survivors after a death by suicide.

Survivors need to receive the greatest gentle compassion for their soul state and not be expected to just "get on with life." Religious sacraments, journaling, gardening, time in nature, music, artistic activities and healthy work, can all be valuable steps in healing. It is extremely helpful to stay in contact with survivors after the first flurry around a death has come and gone. It is very important for them to have friends with whom they can continue to talk about the death and their precious relationship to the loved one who has passed on. They will be especially grateful when you can remember anniversaries, and help keep the good memories of their loved ones integrated as a natural part of life.

Final Thoughts

As stated before, to do all these things for a death at home requires a group of people willing to help when needed and at least a few with full awareness of what needs to be done. This extensive ritual may not be possible or appropriate in many cases. What is practical, good and right for any person and their family is what needs to be done. But regardless of circumstances, of religious views, traditions, cultural mores or cultural cynicism, this is a deeply important time for all involved. Contemplation and support of the spiritual destiny and legacy of the dying one, and compassionate support of the survivors, always, always, brings goodness into the universal scheme of life.

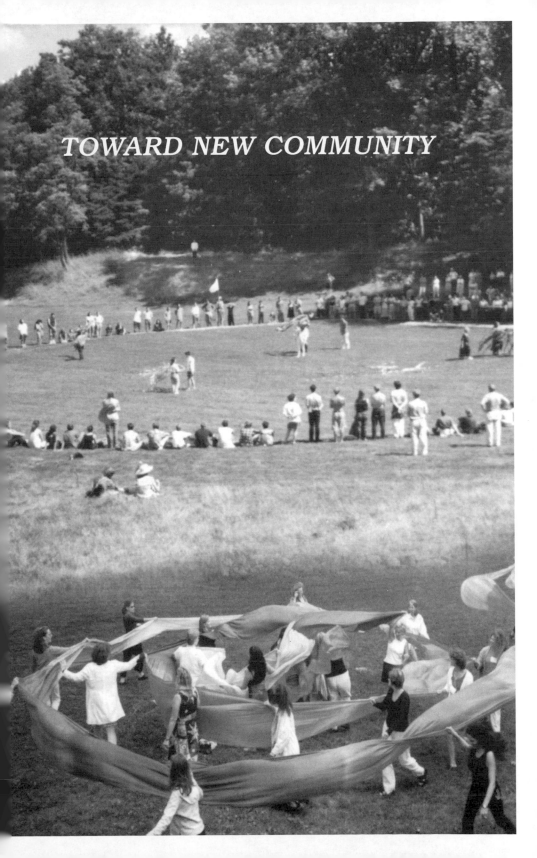

TOWARD NEW COMMUNITY

TOWARD NEW COMMUNITY

When we ponder the mystery of human life, we immediately face the tremendous gulf that exists between our longing for independence and self-realized individuality and our longing to be held and appreciated by a community. On the one hand, we are self-interested and self-serving, keenly aware of our rights, our feelings, our loneliness and isolation. Further, we have well developed critical judgements of others which separates us from them. On the other hand, we want to be accepted and loved. But as modern individuals, we cannot tolerate becoming anonymous, or being subjugated in a group process. Rather, we hope to be a dynamic part of creating new possibilities for things that could not be done alone.

When this dichotomy in our nature becomes evident, we can realize how profoundly death shakes us to bridge these two extremes. It is a bold reminder of our need for one another, our dependence on the efforts of countless hearts and hands for our very existence. It puts us in touch with the core of our being and the deepest questions of our spiritual faith. Death brings us to the hard truth of how we are choosing to live. We must deal with it; a conscious facing of death is a demand of our time. In the end, it is through confronting death that we are truly and fully able to live our lives.

When we experience deaths in our life, we can become focused again and awake to our humanity, mindful of the brevity of life, pulled from our materialistic muddlings and back to the higher priorities of a meaningful life. The sorrow and pain of our loss can strip us of our gratuitous persona, our masks, and our facades. The barriers we use to shield ourselves from others can be laid aside. Here we can become vulnerable and open enough to truly sense and experience others. We can open our hearts to our brothers and sisters in spirit—those not related to us through blood, race, religion, education or social status, but through our *common humanity.*

In the journey of humanity through time we see ever new capacities being forged, be they in the outer mastery of fire and tools, or the inner journey of the soul and spirit. In every age there are those, both godlike and human, who pioneer a path, and forge new enobled soul qualities for all the human race. Most often it has been through the fire of suffering and the courageous and creative transformation of life's challenges that such individuals have shown the way for posterity.

In the last hundred years, we have also plumbed the lower recesses of the human soul, seeking awareness of the realms of the unconscious.

Certain aspects of that journey have been a necessity too, in order to face, name, and own what lurks there in our own being, so that it cannot manipulate us undetected from the shadows. Transformation at this soul level assumes heroic proportions. It is the battle for new capacities in our time; and the self-knowledge won in the process is a deed of tremendous benefit not only for the individual, but for the whole community and the progress of humanity. Sadly, we know of many who have not been able to win their freedom, but are driven by the powerful forces of the lower soul nature.

But there is always help when it is asked for, and we do have choices. As modern self-directing, conscious individuals we can ask ourselves, Where we are choosing to give the most precious possessions we have to give—our attention, our interest, our time, our vitality, our commitment and our love? Are we directing these gifts toward a healthy body, a rich soul, an open inquiring mind, an enlivened spirit, deepened relationships, caring for loved ones, and toward the good of the greater community?

Today we have opportunities to transform, develop, discipline, and direct our soul forces unlike at any time before in world history. This is because we have developed to a point where we can make conscious choices. It is also because so many individuals have walked the path and showed a way that we may follow. We can stand in awe before the collective deeds for the good throughout history that have led human evolution toward individuality, choice and freedom—and toward a new conscious community where we recognize one another as spiritual individualities.

Consider some of the gifts we are heir to, some of the possibilities for our own development, because Zarathustra brought light into the powers of darkness, because Krishna counseled Arjuna that there is immortal life beyond the physical realm, because Abraham brought wisdom, because Moses brought the Law and Confucius brought sagacity, because Taliesin, the Celtic bard, sang of this world and the next and Bride guarded the holy flame. Buddha brought compassion, Plato brought philosophy, and Aristotle formed human thought to understand the world. Because Christ lived and Mary suffered the death of her son, because Paul preached, and Manu transformed evil. Because St. Francis suffered and loved the world and Parsifal, dumb and stumbling, eventually triumphed on the search for the Grail, and the Sufi mystic, Rumi, sang his poetry of life. Because Degandawidah, the Iroquois holy man, forged the six nations with the law of peace, Joan of Arc followed the angel Michael and wielded her sword of courage, Shakespeare lifted the soul's journey to winged words, Rembrandt and Raphael held a paint brush and Beethoven wrote the Ninth symphony. Because George Washington prayed at Valley Forge, Harriet Tubman saved her people and Lincoln championed their cause, because Bahaullah brought a gentle Bahai faith, because Ralph Waldo Emerson's mother raised a man who would be an eloquent moral genius, because Helen Keller and Annie Sullivan shone their spirit light to millions, because the Wright brothers lifted their creation aloft despite gravity, because Pasteur saw keenly and practiced his science, because Albert Schweitzer served in Africa, because Anne Frank awakened to life amidst darkness, and Ghandi fasted and brought nonviolence to a nation. Carl Jung honored the human soul and Rudolf Steiner showed the way to spirit. Because Thich Nhat Hanh and the Dalai Lama counsel mindfulness, because Mother Hale loves and redeems drug babies, because Martin Luther King, Jr. and Peace Pilgrim walked the nation for civil rights and peace and Mother Teresa served the dying.

And there are countless more, millions more, both famous and unremembered—a veritable nation of souls, brothers and sisters whose scope and breadth of deeds of courage, inspiration, and transformation cover the sweep of history and embrace us all with their universality. They have woven shimmering, eternal, golden threads through the thick, ponderous, and bloodied tapestry of human world history.

In the holy death of Christ, which affected the world as no other death has, there is a defining, founding moment for new community on earth. It is meant for all humanity, not just those who profess the Christian faith. Near the end of the agony, the great Being of light and compassion looked down from the cross to the up turned, sorrow-filled faces of the few who remained faithful to the last, including his mother and his beloved disciple, John. With His last words, He said to his mother, "Woman, behold thy son," and, to John, "Behold thy mother." The Gospel goes on to tell us, "And from that hour the disciple took her unto his own home." (John 19: 26-27). This is the founding for new community, given at the threshold of death, at the foot of the cross. The last commandment of Christ is to love one another as your own, not just those related by common blood. This is exemplified in the life of Mother Teresa who saw and served the light of the spirit in everyone she met.

Christ is a pure universal being of light who had no need to go through death. Yet He chose to walk with humanity through death, through sacrifice, loneliness and persecution in order to place into the stream of human evolution new powers of healing, forgiveness, resurrection, and love. Because of this deed these capacities can be awakened ever anew in our own souls and spirits.

Ultimately, good must be done. When our human thoughts, feelings, and behavior are merely reactions to our world, they cannot generate new powers. Courage, generosity, and love do not exist in us, or in the world, until we create them with the power of our own conscience and will. It is a creative act of the highest order and one to be entered into daily—to pledge one's will to the good, to give service to others. Death is around us as a reminder of the brevity of our time to do so. When our conscience speaks and we follow with action it becomes a sacred alchemy that creates the gold of moral powers in the soul. We become sun-like within and the soul and spirit are then capable of shedding warmth and light and generating new life in all those we meet.

Our collective legacy of great human gifts and deeds from the whole world has expanded our soul possibilities to the very stars. They shine from the past, into the present and light the way to the future with the brilliance of countless rays of light, light pooled into a common life-giving sun that shines upon us all. They have expanded our possibilities to the greatest limits, giving us challenge and hope. Christopher Fry writes of this eloquently in his classic poem that follows:

This chapter was written in memorium for those who died in the United States, September, 11, 2001.

From "A SLEEP OF PRISONERS"

Good has no fear

Good is itself, whatever comes.

It grow, and wakes, and bravely

Persuades, beyond all tilt of wrong:

Stronger than anger, wiser than strategy,

Enough to subdue cities and men

If we believe it with a long courage of truth

The human heart can go to the lengths of God.

Dark and cold we may be, but this

Is no winter now. The frozen misery

Of centuries breaks, cracks, begins to move;

The thunder is the thunder of the floes,

The thaw, the flood, the upstart Spring.

Thank God our time is now when wrong

Comes up to face us everywhere.

Never to leave us till we take,

The longest stride of soul men ever took.

Affairs are now soul size

The enterprise

Is exploration into God

Where are you making for? It takes

So many thousand years to wake,

But will you wake for pity's sake?

WHY THERE HAS TO BE A BETTER WAY

The Story of Luz

This is a story of two women who "were there" at a time of greatest need and who came when there was no one else to help. They had been concerned for some time about finding better ways to support families when death occurs and had recently pioneered a community service business to offer aid.

They had just begun their work when they got a call from a mother frantic with grief and pleading with them for help. Her twenty-year-old daughter had just died from a drug overdose. The body was at the coroner's. The mother was desperate to be with her daughter, but the coroner was in no hurry to deal with the matter. The funeral homes weren't interested in the case because the mother was an indigent and there was no money involved.

Further questioning revealed that the mother was virtually homeless, living in a small room with several other people. All her worldly possessions were in an eight-by-twelve storage locker on the edge of town. She was near hysteria with shock and grief, pouring out her anguish in great wails of mourning. There was no place to bring the body so she could have some time for closure. The two women were filled with compassion for her ordeal, but reluctant to bring the body to their own homes. Their business was just in the fledgling stages, and they could not risk any negative publicity.

Finally the mother pleaded with them to bring her daughter's body to the storage unit. Realizing there really wasn't any other alternative, the women agreed. Armed with the proper paper work, they picked up her remains in a zippered body bag at the coroner's facility and put it in the back of their van. Driving through the city streets, entering the storage facilities, winding down the narrow alleys to find the right storage garage was tension-filled work. All the time they feared witnesses to the process who might hinder the work and bring difficult repercussions. Nonetheless, they were also determined they were going to help this deserted and sorrowing mother. At the unit, the mother was waiting for them alone, her face anxious and hopeful.

But a further trauma awaited. The body had been put into the bag upside down. They had expected to just unzipper it part way to reveal the girl's face. Instead they had to open the bag at the feet, slowly revealing her full young form, beautiful, naked, and scarred with the slashes of the autopsy. But an amazing thing happened. As soon as the mother could see and touch her daughter's body, no matter how mutilated, she became instantly calm. She touched, she crooned, she nurtured. She went into the storage locker and brought out her daughter's baby clothes, baby shoes, her first blankets and little toys, her school pictures, and laid them near the still form. She touched her daughter's face with adoration and showed the women the beautiful color of her eyes.

What followed was just as poignant. Inside the storage unit, the mother had pushed back boxes and furniture. There at the entrance she had gathered colorful scarves, pictures, candles, and flowers, and had made two shrines: one to Buddha, and one to Christ. The two women were overcome with the mother's tender, loving efforts to create beauty for her daughter's passage.

So it came to pass, before the journey to the crematorium, for a few brief moments, a storage unit was a holy cathedral in a service attended by three women and the soul of another close by in spirit. I am confident it was a service no less attended by angels than the most glorious offering in a church that seats a thousand. Here a heart-felt, sacred ritual created by a sorrowing mother for the passing of her beautiful, young daughter was played out as she lifted her prayers to all the gods of universal goodness. It became an act of consecration that must have glowed in heaven on behalf of the lonely and abandoned everywhere.

Thank goodness those two brave women were there for the mother at this transition. Our mainstream ways of deathcare have too often failed to give grieving families humane choices to care for their loved ones. There has to be a better way.

CIRCLES IN THE COMMUNITY OF LIFE

Linda and Kirsten

This is a story of community—a weaving between families, between people who suffered the hardest kind of loss and those who helped them, and a weaving with the guiding inspiration of loved ones who have crossed the threshold. Mostly it is my story about Linda, who is my friend. But in actuality the whole story involves a very large circle of people and each one of them could add a special chapter to this account to create a most extraordinary volume of community life.

Linda, a tall, vivacious woman, worked as a teacher and therapist. Her husband Paul Bergh, a social worker, was a robust bear of a man with a warm humor and a passionate love of language, literature and music. Both Linda and Paul took great delight in their lively and talented only child, Kirsten. They also shared an impulse for a communal life as did some of their best friends, Patrick and Diana O'Brien, who had one young daughter, Molly. Before marriage, all these individuals had lived in various communal situations. Nevertheless, it is doubtful that they would have taken the step they did to create conscious community, by purchasing a home together, had it not been for the insistence of their daughters. Kirsten and Molly wanted the experience of sisters, though Molly was almost two years younger than Kirsten. So the two sets of parents took the optimistic steps to buy a pleasant old home in Minneapolis together, with the Bergh family living upstairs, and the O'Briens downstairs. Not long into the arrangement, Linda and Diana realized they had a special sisterhood as well. Both women would later remember the soul moment when they made an unspoken, but mutually acknowledged, commitment to be there for one another through whatever life would bring. Diana remembers thinking at the time, "Okay, here we go." Little did she know then, how profound that pledge of support would prove to be in the years to come.

There was another family who would also share destiny with the Berghs in ways neither family could have anticipated. Marianne and Dennis Dietzel had three children, two sons and a daughter, Nina, who was one of Kirsten's closest friends. The three families all enjoyed outdoor life, had many rich cultural interests and were committed to an international Waldorf education for their daughters. And all three of the girls, Kirsten, Nina and Molly, were woven in each others lives, finding in one another a sisterhood they had always wanted.

When Kirsten turned fourteen, Linda and Paul decided they would spend a year abroad in France. There Kirsten's artistic talents blossomed while attending a French Waldorf school and taking painting lessons. Linda and Paul took jobs as house parents and teachers in a small group home for disturbed adolescents. Though the work was intense, the three of them were able to enjoy weekends exploring the country with treks to old churches and museums, hiking and biking in the pastoral countryside, savoring French breads and cheeses and making new friends. Most of all, they enjoyed each other, little realizing they were condensing memories for a lifetime into these few months.

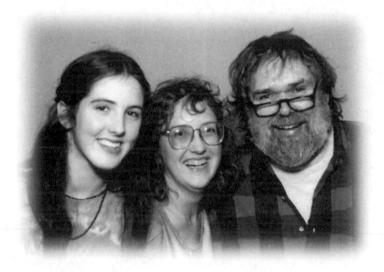

A year after they returned home, Paul suffered a cardiac arrest and quickly lapsed into a coma. At the hospital, Kirsten stayed long hours by his side, sobbing, holding his hand, pleading for him to stay, and singing every song she and her father had ever sung until she was breathless with exhaustion. Linda took her daughter for a long walk and they shared their grief and tried to imagine a future without Paul. Afterward as they gathered in the hospital corridor with Dianna and Molly, the doctor gave them the hard news that Paul would not recover. Closing the door of the small windowless waiting room of the ICU unit, the four women stood in a circle, hugging, weeping, and keening their loss. Then shouldering the hard reality of Paul's passing, they resolved together to create a loving space to help Paul let go. As they re-entered the intensive care room and gathered around his bed, Paul, even through a deep coma, was smiling. They all saw it.

During this time, friends had flocked to the hospital to be with Paul. Hospital rules only allowed biological relatives to visit. So Linda identified everyone who came as family, Paul's or her brothers and sisters. They were family—"soul" family. They needed to be there. When the hospital staff finally figured out what was happening, they let it go. A friend called to the hospital and asked Linda what message she would like to go out to the community. With a steady voice, Linda replied, "I want people to help him cross over. That is the message." Ultimately, wife and daughter together with their soul family friends, gathered around Paul's bed and sang him across the threshold as he died. Some of the nurses, deeply moved, later told them how they wished everyone there could die that way.

From the moment of Paul's death, Linda, Diana and Patrick and the others were united with one overwhelming resolve—they wanted Paul home. And they wanted him accompanied by one of them at each step of the way. It was new experience for everyone. Patrick found a crematorium where they would let the family wash and prepare the body. He rode in the funeral home vehicle to the place, while Dennis, after many phone calls, finally found dry ice at a store with fishing supplies. Dennis, Diana and Linda washed and prepared Paul's body together. It was intense, fulfilling, ground breaking experience for each of them. Paul's death would be the first in that community with a three day vigil at home. They laid his body in the casket and placed it in a small, unadorned, meditation room that Paul had carefully built. Some of those who came to honor Paul and the family were at first apprehensive about seeing him in this intimate setting, without the formality of a funeral home. But afterward, many stated they were amazed at the unanticipated feelings of deep peace they experienced in that quiet and unhurried sacred space. Paul's transition would begin an awareness of new ways to work with death that still reverberates through the wider community, affecting the choices many have since made about their own deaths.

Kirsten poured her sorrow for her father's passing into her poetry and journals, and her loss brought her even closer to her best friends, Nina and Molly. When the three girls heard about a small Waldorf youth conference for young adults, they all wanted to go even though they were still in high school. They wrote letters together petitioning to attend. They were accepted, and were the youngest participants there. Nina was seventeen, Kirsten, sixteen, and Molly almost fifteen. Kirsten and Nina came home inspired to again go to a Waldorf school and further experience the education they had loved when they were young. Molly was already planning a year abroad in a Waldorf school in France. As there was no Waldorf high school in Minneapolis where they lived, they begged their parents to let them enroll in one in New York state. For Linda, and for Nina's parents, Marianne and Dennis, it was a hard decision to let their children go away to a school a thousand miles from home. But all the parents were committed to support-ing their daughters' unfolding hopes and dreams. The girls went off in high spirits and Linda went to join them for the Thanksgiving holidays.

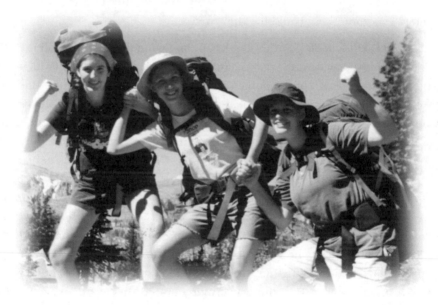

Kirsten, Molly, and Nina

The reunion was joyful. With adolescent verve, Kirsten and Nina shared all their new experiences, for they both had very quickly become a dynamic part the community, known for their enthusiasm and love for their friends, their studies, life in general, and especially for their devotion to one another. On the day after Thanksgiving, Linda and the two girls set off gaily for a shopping trip. Kirsten was driving as they traveled over the country roads toward town, chatting happily together. On a curve, the car hit invisible black ice and slid into the path of an on-coming truck. The girls were killed instantly, the impact thrusting Kirsten into Nina's arms as they died together. Linda, severely injured, was rushed to a nearby hospital.

The school community, shocked and stunned like all of us who knew them, immediately rallied. There was no question they wanted to provide the care needed for Nina and Kirsten themselves. A group of families closest to the girls quickly arranged for the heartbreaking call to Nina's parents, for the care of the girls' bodies and for someone to be with Linda. One of the families offered their home for the vigil. A man who had not even known the girls made the coffins. He had two daughters of his own.

In the living room of the home, the girls were laid in the hastily and carefully made caskets. Nina, who was fair, wore a beautiful white peasant blouse and skirt. In the summer Nina had requested a special white tiered skirt and she and her mother had selected the material and began to sew it together. Marianne finished it, and sent it with Molly, who flew out to be with the girls for Nina's birthday. Kirsten lay with her lustrous black tresses softly about her face, clad in a dark green linen blouse, a long colorful skirt and the shadow of a dark wound across her lovely brow. In death as in life, the girls were side by side, heart wrenching in their youthful beauty.

Over the next days, classmates, friends, and Nina's parents and family streamed in and out of the room, weeping, hugging, singing, consoling, praying and struggling to come to terms with the tragedy. Patrick, Diana and Molly came too, once again taking the responsibilities of close "soul" family. After the funeral service, they were the ones who accompanied the girls' bodies to the crematorium. Bravely young Molly, who had just lost her two most cherished friends, took that long journey too. Molly had just completed a school assignment to write about a poet and had chosen Kirsten. With the admiration of a devoted younger sister, she had memorialized Kirsten's poetry in a booklet, a tribute which Kirsten had just received the night before she died.

In the hospital miles away, Linda lay, with her body broken and her face shattered from the forehead down. The initial surgery to rebuild the twenty eight broken bones in her face took fourteen hours. Her jaw was wired closed. The sight in one eye was gone. Ultimately six more surgeries would be required to successfully create a nose so she could breathe well.

Hovering on the edge of life, Linda was sustained by community friends. Someone from the girl's school was with her constantly until two of her close professional friends, Larry and Carol, a psychiatrist and psychiatric nurse, arrived to stay with her. They had planned to take a vacation the day of the accident but had unexplained feelings of uneasiness all morning. When the news came, they flew immediately to Linda's side and remained with her day and night for the first week. Friends all over the country began to pray for her freedom to make the choice that was rightly hers, to go or to remain on earth now that her husband and child were gone. Many were later surprised to find they had been holding her with the same prayer.

Flying out just after an intense ice storm, Patrick and Diana came to the hospital to see Linda. As she walked into the room, Diana was amazed to feel Linda's lack of fear in spite of her incredible situation. Yet the anguish was clear for both. Linda could not even cry, for her tear ducts had been destroyed. Whispering through her wired jaw she pleaded to her friend, "Cry for me, cry for both of us, don't hold back. Please go be with Kirsten." Diana, Kirsten's "down-stairs mother", now took up her poignant work from a pledge made long ago, to do what Linda would have done for her daughter and now could not possibly fulfill herself.

After the funeral, Patrick had to fly home to work. Diana and Molly drove back to the school community where they were once again given warm welcome and support. But when Molly left to return to school abroad, it was Diana's lonely task to bring Kirsten's belongings home. Going into Kirsten's room, recognizing all the things she loved; her viola, her books, her poetry, the latest painting, Molly's book of her poetry lying on her bed, the mother's anguish was overwhelming, for herself, for Linda. She knew she could not leave these precious things to the indifferent handling of the airlines. She resolved to carry them all on her own body back home. She would find herself changing planes in Chicago, weighted with the treasured relics, Kirsten's journals, paintings—and her ashes, walking the huge, long cavernous stretches of the airport and suddenly feeling like she had done all this before in some ancient ritual of caring for the dead. The blinking lights of the airport corridors were suddenly surreal as she tried to reconcile her sacred task with this strange, modern setting.

Meanwhile at the hospital, Larry and Carol were constant companions for Linda. They later described Linda's remarkable response to her ordeal. As a psychiatrist, Larry had often worked in emergency rooms situations. He told me he had almost never seen someone like Linda. He described that from the moment she came out of surgery she was in charge. She was clear and resolved, directing her communication through swaths of bandages, a broken body, and a wired jaw. "We entered into a kind of charade," Larry explained. Understanding her need for food or turning was easy. But they went further to her deeper experience of things, communicating intuitively and later with softly whispered requests as Linda learned to speak by covering the tube inserted in her trachea. With a quiet, unwavering persistence, Linda was making sure that she would be a part of the decisions that were affecting her. Larry and Carol were her allies and spokes persons. At Linda's direction, pictures of her before the accident, along with some of Paul and Kirsten, were put up in the room. When any one came to care for her, Larry and Carol introduced them to the "before" Linda, and to her family as well, so that by the time they got to the bed they knew who Paul was, knew about Kirsten, the daughter who had just died, and something about Linda. The nurses were taken beyond their natural empathy for a patient and brought to a "meeting" with this courageous woman for whom they were to render care. Nor did Linda's teaching work stop there. When doctors would make their rounds with students and, as so often happens, lapse into talking about the patient as though she was not really there, Linda would interrupt them and bring them back to center, reminding them that she was a vital and conscious person in the circle.

The hospital gave way before this kind of spiritual authority. When the young people came from Kirsten and Nina's school, they were allowed into the intensive care unit to cluster close around Linda's bed. Without her glasses and only having vision in one eye, she could barely see. She wanted to be sure she could hear every word of the songs the young people had created for the memorial service for the girls. It was a touching sight to see her surrounded by the beautiful earnest young men and women, singing, playing the guitar for her, sharing sorrow and offering hope. Linda later reported she felt so strongly held during these days by all the friends close by, and those who were praying for her across the country.

But there was more. Though Larry and Carol did not necessarily share Linda's spiritual philosophy of life, they found through their faithful vigil of support that they were witness to spiritual care giving that they could not doubt was happening Linda was having recurring visions of radiant beings, like healing sun rays ministering to her during that time. Not only did Linda tell her friends about these care givers from another realm, but they could see her visibly relax, respond and move toward a sense of peace when they were present. These invisible healers would be with her all the first week and as she was flown by air ambulance back to a hospital in her hometown to try, unsuccessfully, to save her eye. Then once home, Linda was immediately surrounded by her home community. Her only brother came for a week and friends flew in from across the country.

With her clear, considerate, yet straightforward way Linda let them know, above all, she did not want to be left alone. She also asked for help to be fed as her arm was broken too. The community responded. Her godchild's mother arranged for shifts to be set up. For the first week, Linda had someone with her all day and all night in her hospital room, and thereafter all during the day. A stream of friends brought organic vegetables and fruits, some donated by the local co-op, to be blended and pureed into nutritious soups by many helpful hands and then fed to her with a syringe through her wired jaw. All this support allowed her to recuperate with fresh healing foods instead the stomach tube that would have otherwise been the source of her nutrition.

Small children of the families would come and sit on the bed and color pictures or sing for her. An understanding and supportive hospital staff allowed local friends and those who flew in from around the country to minister to her undisturbed between hospital routines with prayer, quiet conversation and touching her with healing hands. The nurses and aides would later say they had never experienced such light as when they entered Linda's room.

After six weeks, though still only part way through what would be a long convalescence, Linda left the hospital and returned to her empty home. Though Patrick and Diana, living downstairs, would be steadfastly beside her in the coming months, she had to face the stark quiet, without Paul, and now with the rooms devoid of Kirsten's vibrancy—devoid of the swirling life force of her vivacious, raven-haired daughter who had flung herself into life with passionate ideals, in jeans patched with wild splashes of color, (yet the patches ever so carefully embroidered on the edges); who had wanted to go to Africa to save the animals; who ran barefoot in dew covered grass and climbed up trees and talked to them, and then wrote about it with decisive, sweet and eloquent words in her poetry; who was fervently loyal to her friends and parents; who was bright, merry and deep, like a beautiful bell whose very sound quickens the heart.

Certainly the question was always there that Linda must have asked countless times, "Why did she survive the accident?" How could she go on? What was there to live for? No husband, no child, no parents. She literally had to look out at the world through an entirely different face. What could the future possibly hold?

But never did her courage fail her, and this has made all the difference.

What distinguished her response to this ultimate tragedy has been her openness—her willingness **to walk into the pain.** Linda never gave up, and she felt through it all it was not her time to die. She drank the full bitter cup, and deep in her soul she resolved not to become the bitterness.

Once at home, Linda read her daughter's private journals for the first time. She found not only uplifting poetry, but beautifully drawn figures filled with joyful vitality. She was astounded to find some were almost identical to the vibrant, healing spiritual beings she had experienced in the first days after the accident. Longing to share the poetry and art with all who had been close to Kirsten became a mission for her and with the help of a friend she published it in a book *She Who Would Draw Flowers.** She gave the book to Kirsten and Nina's classmates to help them with the struggle and loss they were going through. Then she joined them in planting a tree and flowers at the accident site. Both she and Nina's parents attended the graduations of their daughters' classes.

Linda took the poetry book into high school classes, (as did other teachers across the country), where it spoke to the hearts of countless young people who embraced Kirsten as their own. When using Kirsten's poetry to help an inner city high school class cope with loss, a student asked her, "Why do you do this when it makes you sad?" Linda quietly replied, "I've vowed never to run away from this. And because of it I have met you, and now something new can happen."

Then, much later, she took the steps to reach the driver of the truck. She had wanted to give him support, knowing he had suffered too. She was finally able to write him a letter. He was astounded to hear from her. She assured him she was slowly healing her body and her heart. Through letters, and then phone calls, she reassured him he was not held with anything but caring thoughts. Six months later they met each other face to face, and were able to further loosen the bindings of grief from their destiny encounter.

The summer following the accident, I urged Linda to attend a large international youth conference that Kirsten and Nina would surely have attended had they been here. She was still fragile in her recovery process, yet longed to be there. In the end, she came, as did Nina's mother and father, these three caring, grieving parents, who still wanted to be offering support for other young people. For those of us who knew the story, it was heart rending to see Linda standing at the doorway of the big meeting hall as the young people left for lunch break, handing each one a copy of Kirsten's book of poetry with a warm look and a smile. The next day, a young woman placed the book in the open space in the center of the concentric circles of participants (250 youth and elders) as they were engaged in deep and meaningful conversation. As she laid it on the floor into a pool of sunlight that streamed through the tall stately windows of the hall, she spoke out in a clear, vibrant voice, "This belongs here—in the center."

Linda returned home after the youth conference deeply fulfilled at having shared Kirsten and Nina's story and the book of poetry with such a responsive group of young people. But after being with the girls' contemporaries, new waves of grief and loss swept over her. Further, in the midst of her anguish, she had to endure new bouts of pain from the seemingly endless surgeries and constant work to heal her body. Through this time she was steadied and held by the faithful support of friends, listening, helping with her appointments, her food, and therapies. She worked toward healing through art and writing, through the beauty of nature, her daily meditative spiritual practice, and the ephemeral sense of Paul's and Kirsten's continuing presence.

Yet the pain that comes with such loss and grief is inevitably the eye of the needle we have to go through alone. While the community surrounded her in every possible way with concern and support, the caring must have seemed at times to come from far away, like earnest voices calling up to someone high on a mountain, alone in the rarified winds and full glare of the sun. Often in those first three years, Linda's voice came to us from a place I have come to call "behind the veil." It is a phrase I feel describes a place where we can inwardly move after the shocking loss of a loved one. It is part way into another world. Her voice then was often very soft and wrought with compassion. But perhaps through her sorrow and loneliness she was more accompanied than she knew and more than we realized. For all the obvious pain, there was an aura about her.

Linda's gratitude and openness to receive support helped create some beautiful, deeply human meetings. Her honesty engendered a rare sense of freedom and inspiration for others to be with her. During the long months of her recuperation, countless visitors would come to see her. After they asked about her and received her candid replies about her frustration or crankiness, or pain or joy, she would then ask about their lives. The stories wove back and forth in human communion, mutual stories of struggle, sadness, secretly held griefs, joys and triumphs, shared in the ebb and flow of tears and laughter. It was a safe and gentle space where sorrows, hopes and challenges could be lifted and released again into the stream of life, the stream of healing and love. Linda would often tell me of that deep truth—by giving we receive and by receiving we give.

As she went through the long recovery process, often just getting through from one day to the next, Linda also came to realize just how greatly she had been surrounded by caring friends. In reflecting back with others on all that occurred in those intense life changing days, a picture of the concentric circles of community support around her has emerged in ever greater detail. Close by were her spiritual soul families who gave her daily, on going support. Then there were Kirsten and Nina's school communities, both at home and where they died, selflessly contributing when the need was so immediate, as well as all the friends, family and colleagues across the country. Diana, who was at the center of caring around Linda, described how she was constantly amazed by all the many acts of kindness that flowed into that space of need. The uplifting hope created by that caring is just as fresh and vibrant today as the day when the help was given. Linda and everyone involved have experienced a vital deepening of community connections; all the compassionate deeds interweaving with the encircling guiding warmth of angels and loved ones from the other side, creating the spiritual substance that unites heaven and earth, life and love.

We cannot truly know the full answer to the question of why Linda survived when all her family was gone. Certainly she brought Kirsten's enlivening words of poetry to many people. In the face of the ultimate tragedies, she has chosen to keep on living, to stay open to all life offers. Countless people have been inspired, uplifted and aided in re-focusing their lives through her example that the hardest life challenges can be met and transformed. She is a testimony of hope. Happily, her personal life continues to improve. She could always sing; now she can once again dance as well, and has a new partner to love. My view is that she has been able to say "Yes" to life, even with a heart hollowed with sorrow and that has allowed the space to be filled with a spiritual light she can bring to others. She has walked the path of sorrow, courage, forgiveness, and renewed love for all.

Linda once quietly shared with me an experience she had when Larry and Carol took her for a return trip to France, and visited some of the places where she and her family had spent their last year together. In a little town, in a small, old, stone church, she sat alone before a statue of a primitive black madonna. Such ancient and revered statues are reminders of the ever-

195

lasting nurturing maternal power of the universe. They can inspire a deep transformative peace. There in a quiet moment, Linda felt a surrounding spiritual presence. Then she experienced a feeling like the softness of a mantle being laid over her shoulders, giving her a sense of being held and comforted in a profoundly gentle way.

It is not hard for me to imagine her being so blessed. I sense that such an experience can not only be a sign of divine love and protection, but also a mantle of acknowledgement. Such individuals as Linda, and those who helped her, are doing the work of the divine mother, the eternal feminine on earth, for they are bringing deeds of healing warmth and love into a world that desperately needs it.

With her body well recovered and again four square and feisty, Linda emphatically tells me not to describe her in holy terms stating she is "all too human." She is right, of course. But human and holy is just what we all are, and that is just the marvel of it all. How ordinary and human we are, yet what universal divinity we manifest when we act with love in serving and caring for one another. It is the crowning essence of community life. When individuals unite their highest and holiest they can create undreamed of power to transform the world for the good.

Linda, and all of us who know her, continue to marvel at the events which are still unfolding from the transitions of Paul, Kirsten, and Nina. Along with recurring grief, always to be met and borne again and lifted anew, have also come countless healings and community initiatives following in the wake of these destinies. Nina's mother, Marianne, quietly began a weekly group to remember the girls and other loved ones on the other side, and to read together for them. That work now reaches wide circles and inspires many to take up further threshold work. Like Kirsten's book of poetry lying in a pool of sunlight at the youth conference and reaching out to the surrounding circles of those meeting there, it is amazing how the vitality and spirit of Paul and the girls keeps touching and inspiring so many people's lives. The interweaving among those on earth and those in spirit have created a web of community that keeps expanding to new levels of wonder and joy. They are like endless ripples from a pebble dropped in a beautiful pond, moving out through the depths of suffering and transformation in ever widening circles of radiant light, reflecting the spiritual essence of the sun into our lives.

She Who Would Draw Flowers, Kirsten Savitri Bergh, is available through Linda Bergh, 4315 Xerxes Ave. S., Minneapolis, Minn. 55410, E mail, Lindabergh @ AOL.com, or Anthroposophical Press 1-800-856-8664.

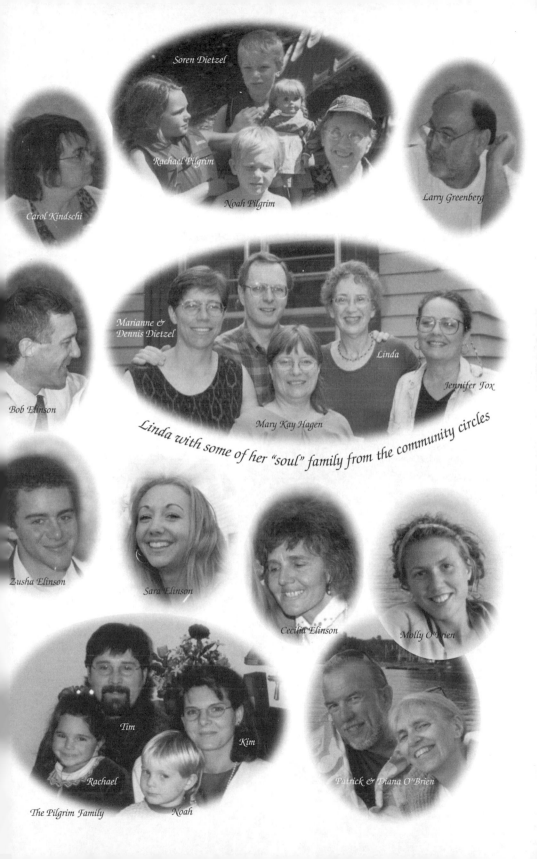

Soren Dietzel

Rachael Pilgrim

Noah Pilgrim

Carol Kindschi

Larry Greenberg

Marianne &
Dennis Dietzel

Linda

Jennifer Fox

Bob Elinson

Mary Kay Hagen

Linda with some of her "soul" family from the community circles

Zusha Elinson

Sara Elinson

Cecilia Elinson

Molly O'Brien

Tim

Kim

Rachael

Noah

The Pilgrim Family

Patrick & Diana O'Brien

FOR YOU, PAPA

I thought I heard your footsteps
running toward me,
disturbing the stones.
But when I opened my eyes,
I saw it was only the waves,
Pulling and swirling like hands.

I thought I felt your smile,
Warm and loving upon my face.
But when I opened my eyes,
I saw it was only the sun,
Beaming at me from across the water.

I thought I heard you
Whisper my name.
But when I opened my eyes,
I realized it was only the wind
Playing in my hair.

I thought I felt you
Softly kiss my cheek.
But when I opened my
eyes,
I saw it was only a leaf
Caressing me with gentle
strokes.

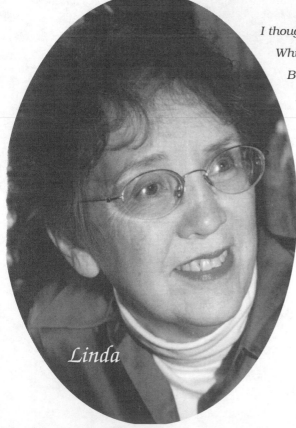

Linda

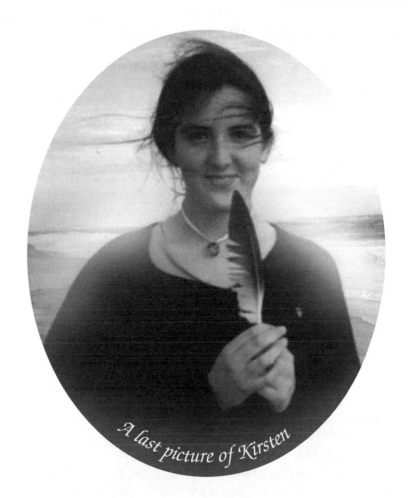

A last picture of Kirsten

And then I felt your love
In and all around me.
Powerful, yet gentle like the waves,
Warm and shining like the sun,
Soft yet strong like the wind,
Tender and alive like the leaves.
And I didn't even have
To open my eyes.
I knew you were there.

Kirsten Savitri Bergh

THE MAJOR EVENT OF KIM'S TRANSITION

The Gift of His Dying

The community was on hand, in force, for Kim's exodus to the spiritual world, and it was an event none of us will ever forget. Maulsby "Kim" Kimball and his wife, Ilse, were two fascinating characters in our town and, in their golden years, remained burnished with a lively social light that kept clusters of people around them. There were friends and helpers to attend to Ilse (who was in a wheelchair for five years), to join them both for rounds of parties and celebrations for their birthdays and high festival days, and to gather with them for meetings of study and sharing spiritual work. Papa Kim, as he was known to many, was a painter, a teacher, and counselor to a large group of people, ecumenically gathered from all walks of life.

These two, Ilse and Kim, managed transitions back to the spiritual world that would be the envy of people who had extensive personal family to care for them. They had none. Though well into their eighties, they stayed at home for their final years, with virtually no hospital stints of any duration. Though Kim had bone cancer, he was able to fulfill his pledge to care for his beloved Ilse, and then cross over himself five months later. Both of them died at home and were cared for by the community, their "spiritual" family.

For me, the one who attended Kim at his transition, his death was one of the most special gifts I have ever received. It was an exalted spiritual experience, truly sublime. What then followed was one of the most ludicrous last acts I have ever witnessed, without doubt the epitome of "from the sublime to the ridiculous." But Kim was a great soul who encompassed both these polarities, and everything in between, in his spacious personality. In retrospect, it all seemed to be in character.

Kim was born into a prominent, cultured family on the East Coast, a precocious child who would become a man of enormous intelligence, with an imposing brow, a remarkable nose, and big, china-blue eyes that he used to great advantage. He had an extraordinary wit and a dedicated path of spiritual work.

To say that Kim was an *enfant terrible* as a child, would be to put it mildly. In grammar school, he would lie insolently on his back on the floor and spout the correct answers to the teacher's questions, whether asked or not. These were delivered with a heavy lisp for which he was constantly teased. He was sent home again and again for being incorrigible. For punishment, his parents would banish him to the spacious and beautiful upstairs art, music, and play studio they had designed for their four extraordinarily talented children. But there he only rejoiced in his hours alone, and the opportunity to give free rein to his boundless imagination. The parents eventually withdrew Kim from school and started their own program, hiring teachers with innovative ways to teach their four children and other such creative souls. His younger sister, Emily, whom he both protected and teased unmercifully, was devoted to him.

Kim's attorney father, a gifted musician, wanted Kim to follow him into a law career, but it became quite clear that that wasn't going to happen. So the father challenged Kim that if he was going to be an artist, he had better be a good one, and not add any more mediocre art to the world. He did become a gifted artist, internationally known for his seascapes and beautiful paintings of spiritual subjects, executed in brilliant, flowing colors. As a young adult, he taught art in a prestigious boys' school.

Though he carved out a successful career, Kim did not marry. Then when he was nearly fifty, he became enamored of a diminutive firebrand of a woman, with snapping dark eyes, from an aristocratic family in Vienna. She was a teacher of eurythmy, an art of graceful, disciplined movement to make visible the creative power and vitality behind music or the spoken word. She excelled at her work, and was especially known for her enchanting portrayal of elves, sprites, and fairies in the eurythmy productions. The two artists honored one another in a particularly touching relationship and a marriage that lasted over thirty years. They were truly endearing. In old age, Ilse would sometimes sigh passionately that, alas, they had had no babies—but she had taught thousands of little children. Kim would counter with a mild twinkle, "Ilse dear, you were fifty-two when we married!" They were like a knight and his lady. When asked if she missed her home in Europe, Ilse would say, "Kim is my home."

Ilse and Kim were very matter-of-fact in preparing for their transitions. When Kim ordered his casket from us, he requested that it be, "Just like Ilse's, only a little longer, please." As we were working on it, he often inquired about his "sarcophagi," drawling out the last syllable with emphasis, knowing full well the singular form of the word was "sarcophagus"—the type of coffin from the ancient tombs that was also used for initiation ceremonies.

He had planned to come to the ranch to admire the "sarcophagi" but, when his strength failed, I took a photo of it to him. He looked at it with keen interest and great delight. Then with a sparkle in those wonderful blue eyes, he announced. "I believe I'll call it Kimball's hope chest!" Five days later he was laid in it, resplendent in a blue suit, a red cravat, and surrounded by a room filled with vibrant, fluid colors shining from his own wonderful paintings.

Ilse had died in July, five months before Kim would cross over. As December came that year, we knew it would be Kim's first Christmas without his beloved wife, so my daughter, Lauren, and I, along with her little three-year-old girl, Gabrielle, bought him a Christmas tree. We decorated it and celebrated the second Sunday of Advent with him, singing and lighting candles together. He sat there with gracious appreciation for the company and the tree glowing gaily with familiar decorations, but it was clear he was not well.

Just that week, Kim had realized he needed full-time help. Up until that time, he had managed extraordinarily well alone. In consultation with the doctor, it was decided that community friends needed to stay with him at night, and I offered to stay an evening the following week, as I had several nights before. The doctor said that, while he was failing rapidly, just when he might go was unknown. I came late Wednesday night, relieving a day helper, to care for him. Kim was in bed, and as the hours passed, he was gradually moving into another consciousness, making restless gestures, and often mumbling incoherently in the process.

My husband came by and joined me for a few minutes. As it turned out, Gordon would be Kim's last visitor. As we came to the bedside, I told him that Gordon was here. Rallying from his labors, Kim managed to pull forth his ready wit; "Oh, the happy husband!" he exclaimed.

Gordon leaned over solicitously, "Kim, are you doing okay?"

"No!" was the emphatic reply.

Somewhat taken back, Gordon shifted nervously. Seeing his discomfort, I encouraged him just to tell Kim good-bye. With that Gordon said, "I'm going to my home in the mountains now, Kim. I'll see you later."

Kim rallied again, now fully present in all his legendary graciousness. In a measured voice, filled with humility and kindness, he told my husband, "Thank you very much for being here just now." I would later tell people it was like an expression of deepest gratitude and appreciation for all the multitudes of friends who had given him help. I felt it was just what he would have told them all.

It was hard to know when he would die. It might be soon, or in two or three days. I looked around the small, cluttered bedroom. Kim used to say his "filing" method was a "piling" method. There were piles of papers and books everywhere. I felt he needed space for dying. Carefully, I removed a clutter of postcards on the wall that were within his range of vision, leaving one, a nativity scene with a sturdy baby Jesus reaching up to a lamb. I placed Leonardo's head of Christ from the Last Supper where he could see it. I tidied the area, but carefully left a square, brown ceramic jug of water on the table. It had always been on his father's desk and was a treasured legacy. Behind the jug, an unframed oil portrait of Kim as a young child, painted by his artistic, semi-invalid mother, leaned against the shelves of books. It was done with obvious love, portraying the sensitive youngster with huge, wistful blue eyes. At the foot of his bed hung a wooden crucifix, a gift from his sister.

Two evenings before, a group of his admirers had come to pay him homage. What a fitting culmination that visit was, honoring the venerable artist for a lifetime of creative work. Kim had managed to get up, dress carefully, and warmly play the host, sharing all the art work in his studio. The friends brought him a beautiful bouquet of magenta roses. The next day the minister came and gave Kim last rites, and in the evening another group of adults and children came and sang Christmas carols for him, which he received with grateful tears.

As the evening now went on, I gave him drops of medicine and kept him warm. His eyes were open, and he lay curled like a child, facing the wall. I brought the roses to him, and held one up before his eyes. He noticed it immediately. Now, as when Gordon had come, he pulled out of his semi-comatose state, like a woman pausing between the contractions of birth. With all his artist's passion for beauty, he beheld the rose and cried, "That is very fine indeed!" Though I didn't know it then, these would be his last words. I took the rose and placed it on the grab bar beside the bed where the blossom would be right before his eyes and placed the rest of the bouquet by the crucifix at the foot of his bed.

The night wore on. Occasionally, he wanted me to hold his hand. But it was also clear when he needed to be alone. I knew I shouldn't disturb him too much. It was his struggle, his labor. He was doing the hard work of dying.

I had had a full day, which ended with a Christmas concert given by my son's school. The children sang the beautiful songs of the coming Christmas season, of Mary and the holy child. Now very tired, for it was after midnight, I knew I needed sleep. Kim's timing was unknown; it could be tomorrow or the next day. I checked him for warmth and water, and then I showered and lay down in the bedroom nearby. I knew we could make it work. I asked the angels to wake me when needed. Then, as surely as a mother wakes through her connection to the child, I got up several times, in between minutes of deeply refreshing sleep. The sleep would prove essential, the only rest I would get for the next twenty hours.

At first when I would check in with him, there seemed no noticeable changes. He struggled and muttered, his eyes transfixed on a faraway place. Then the last time I got up, I could see he clearly had entered another stage. His breath was intense, and he was panting and perspiring. I touched him gently, and felt him respond immediately to my presence. I then began saying the verse we both knew so well from the Foundation Stone Meditation by Rudolf Steiner—the words so especially appropriate to Christmas.

At the turning point of Time

The Spirit-Light of the world

Entered the stream of Earthly evolution

Darkness of Night

Had held its sway;

Day-radiant Light

Poured into the souls of men;

Light that gives Warmth

To simple Shepherds' hearts.

Light that enlightens

The wise Heads of kings.

O Light Divine,

O Sun of Christ!

Warm Thou

Our Hearts,

Enlighten Thou

Our Heads

That good may become

What from our Hearts we would found

And from our Heads direct,

With single purpose.

As the verse unfolded, Kim visibly relaxed, his breath lost the frantic quality and became slower and calmer. Several times I slowly repeated the words, "Christ in you" to him. I began another verse we both knew well. Then something changed. It was as though we both took a step toward the threshold, expanded out, up and beyond, not of this world. Yet we were gently held by a ringing silence and a spiritual presence that was filling the room.

It became very clear that Kim was dying. At the same time, I realized he was responding utterly and completely to the timeless, sacred words. We were uniting in a tremendous work together. With each sentence, his breath became noticeably calmer and more rhythmic; we were in perfect synchronization, in perfect willed harmony. It was nothing personal. I was only a vehicle through which the words could flow. The great "No!" of his agonizing struggle in the earlier hours was changing, transforming, becoming a committed and triumphant, "Yes!" As I ended the verse, I held my breath, thinking this might be the moment, but, no, not just yet.

Aided by powers beyond the physical realm, I felt we were lifted to another plane, wrapped in timelessness, alone and everywhere, at once at the center and at the periphery. I sensed accompaniment, first by Ilse, standing by with all her love for the essence of the word. It was as though she willed her love through me to assist her husband's homecoming. And I felt more, there seemed to be a veritable heavenly host surrounding us and preparing to welcome Kim.

I touched his shoulder, wanting him to be as conscious as possible for his transition. "Christ is waiting," I told him. Then I began reciting the first words of the Gospel of St. John.

> *In the beginning was the Word and the Word was with God,*
> *and the Word was God. The same was in the beginning with God*
> *All things were made through him and without him was*
> *Anything made that was made.*
> *In him was life and life was the light of men*
> *The light shineth in the darkness and the darkness has not*
> *overcome it.*

Kim's breath and each word were completely one. I was witness to soul and spirit, emerging from the body and into the light with the sure grace of a butterfly slipping a cocoon, blended, united in perfect union, wholly one, and holy One, spirit and Word

> *and we have beheld his glory, glory as the only son of the Father,*
> *full of grace and truth.*

Three last breaths with three last words, totally at peace, then the utter silence as Kim was reborn in spirit.

I could hardly believe it. "Just as one might hope," my soul rejoiced, "to die on the word of God!" I was bathed in awe and amazement, for as I shared in his dying I had moved beyond the threshold with him, into hallowed space. "It's happening, it's all happening!" my inner voice exulted, at the same time asking in tremulous wonder, "Am I dying?" So exalted was the moment I was unsure which world I lived in. Every corner of the room was illumined with numinous, supra-earthly light. The silence was filled with the vibrancy of spiritual joy and victory. I wept, tears of wonder, tears of joy, and tears of love for my friend.

I grounded myself with the responsibility to record the time he had crossed over. Holding his watch in my hand I noted it was 3:25 in the morning. A friend told me later the moon just then was in the stars at the foot of the constellation of the Virgin, the divine feminine being of the universe reigning over the moon, as Kim went home to the stars.

I am still in awe at the wondrous timing . . . to die on the holy Word! I felt all Kim's vibrant spirit being permeated and resounding with the Word. I ponder over this with great open questions. I feel these are somehow part of new mysteries, mysteries for the future . . . for me it seems they are also mysteries of Mary . . . Sophia mysteries. Those light-filled moments of Kim's passing live on in my soul with hope and wonder . . .

THE MAJOR EVENT OF KIM'S TRANSITION—ACT TWO

The Community Gathers For Kim

When Maulsby Kimball, a beloved community member crossed over, there was no difficulty in getting community members to come help. They wanted to be there. Even though Kim had just died, they felt the need to be in the presence of his expanding soul and spirit and flocked to his house as soon as the news was out. They all wanted to help and to honor him and this they certainly did.

I was with Kim at his death in the early hours of the morning. There was a quiet and sacred space around his transition, but afterward I knew when I needed to pull myself away from it and call for help to care for his body. Around four o'clock in the morning, I called a young woman, Heidi, who had asked to do threshold work with me. She answered sleepily, and while grateful I had called, was hesitant. I told her Kim had just crossed the threshold I needed some help. She told me it was her little girl's first birthday. "Wonderful!" I exclaimed, and then assured her, "I only need you for about an hour.". So, bless her, she came and helped me bathe and dress him. Kim's spiritual birth, Natalie Jane's first birthday—perfect! Another friend came just then too, and his help was well timed for Kim was not a small man.

In the early morning, my son brought the casket to the house, but he hadn't put in the extra cloths I needed. So I went into the living room and pulled down the red curtains and put them in the bottom of it. Soon three other community friends joined me to help place him in the casket, arrange the paintings, clean and straighten the home, and make all the final arrangements for our esteemed artist friend. It would be exciting for us all to experience the evolution of the beauty of the expression on Kim's face in the coming days of the vigil. Kim was eighty-three when he died, but at the end of the second day, the handsome and unlined face was that a young artist of no more than thirty-five years. It was an incredible, almost unbelievable transformation of his countenance. Several of us were witness to it and felt a sense of wonder that somehow the spirit can make an impression even after death.

But once Kim had crossed over, the grand community drama definitely began. It began with a nervous undertaker, a man for whom this kind of life celebration was much too far beyond his sense of funeral protocol to be able to support it. Kim and Ilse had made all their funeral plans with him years before. They had written out their wishes to die at home, to have a three-day vigil and to be cremated. They had paid for it. It is interesting that the same undertaker had just handled Ilse's death five months before this time, which made his actions when Kim died hard to excuse. Yet he would play his part in the drama to come.

I knew Kim and Ilse had made these arrangements, so I was not concerned about complications. The funeral home would take care of the paper work, the doctor had seen Kim the day before he died and would sign the death certificate, and their official plan was in the mortician's hands. Only it wasn't. Apparently the mortician had filed it away in another one of his facilities and couldn't locate it or recall it. So when I called him late in the morning, he responded in a panicked tone and chastised me for calling so late (Kim had died in the middle of the night) and then went on to ask if I had called the coroner. I didn't see why I should, but told him I would. I did so, and did not encounter any problem with those authorities.

But I didn't get back to the undertaker immediately after calling the coroner because of the many other calls I had to make. In a panic lest he be liable for something, the mortician had called the coroner right after I informed him. Completely counter to Kim's requests, he presented information in a way that would get them involved. He told them we were not relations that were caring for him and that the doctor was not present at the exact moment of death—never mind that doctors are rarely at the bedside when a patient dies a natural death anywhere. I also suspect he was a little annoyed that we insisted on caring for Kim ourselves. Anyway, the coroner's office dispatched a deputy to pick up the body. When someone dies without relatives involved, the coroner can be held responsible to pick up the body and seal the house to prevent vandalism or thievery.

Three of them, a deputy and two helpers, arrived at the house in the afternoon just before I returned from sharing the story of Kim's passing with my teaching colleagues. As I walked in, the elderly minister was just leaving, shaking his head in frustration after having done all he could in the situation to try to convince them this was a religious preference of the deceased.

As I came in, I saw one of the deputy's assistants in the kitchen. He was a thick-necked, beefy man, with a ruddy face. His suit jacket was fastened with one precarious button and stretched over his considerable girth and the coat sleeves rode high above his wrists. Obviously it was a one-size-fits-all official garment grabbed off the rack at the coroner's office. His partner was dressed the same and was of similar stocky size, both were well-built for the task of removing bodies. They looked around, clearly wondering what this job was all about. The deputy coroner was a young black man with a sensitive face and kind eyes. He too, seemed taken aback to find a house full of people. In truth, it was a strange situation indeed: a man who lived alone in this house had just died and he had no relatives, no grieving widow, and no children in need of consolation. Yet here were a dozen people, running about with cheerful demeanor occupying the place!

The young deputy stated his intention to remove the body. Bill, the executor for Kim's estate spoke up first. He was also ex-military, and he had the bearing of authority. He stood toe-to-toe with the deputy firmly stating that he, as executor, was carrying out Kim's orders, and that these orders had been filed with the funeral home, and that there was a doctor to sign the death certificate properly, so there was nothing illegal taking place. In actuality, Bill could not "officially" be the executor until he went to court the next day at ten in the morning and had the title bestowed by a judge, even though it was all written in Kim's will. As this exchange was taking place, Bill's attractive wife, with a warm, mediating smile, began the first of many phone calls to try to reach Kim's only close blood relative, his sister Emily, who lived in Connecticut. If Emily could sanction what was happening, the body could remain. There was no answer. The coffin bearers looked around impatiently and shifted from one foot to the other.

The coroner stated again that he would have to take the body away. The ex-army captain argued—vehemently. As things got intense, a hospitable, soft-spoken community member, Jennifer, now took her moment on stage. She felt we had hardly met this group with appropriate courtesy and she now offered everyone tea, which she graciously served all around. The coffin bearers, obviously ill at ease, sat down on the couch, awkwardly holding the delicate tea cups. Yet they were somewhat resigned that this odd assignment was going to take a while.

During the initial exchange, three of us huddled in a corner to confer on strategy. One was an imposing woman who was a building contractor. She was well over six feet tall and somewhat fearless and aggressive in her manner. An ardent friend of the Kimballs, like all of us present, she now stated she would be quite willing to chain herself to the casket to prevent them from taking it away. The other woman, an attorney's wife, helped us weigh this possibility and we decided this was something some of us might well be willing to do. We debated what it might mean in legal and financial repercussions (and for our reputations) if we all went to jail that way. It would certainly make an interesting news story to have several women chained to a casket and taken to the country jail! So this was filed away as a backup plan. While most of us were unaware of it, the attorney's wife then got a call through to her husband and while we prevailed on the home front, his law partner called a judge, who was off duty, and arranged for an injunction to prevent removal of the body for twenty-four hours. This was backup plan B.

All this time during the unfolding saga, the coroner's deputy had not seen the body. It was in the art studio off the living room, and the door had been closed. After several fruitless posturings of threat and counterthreat, while the phone calls continued in an attempt to reach Kim's sister, the gracious lady stepped forward again. It was unseemly that we were deep in discussion about Kim and they had had no introduction to him. She asked the deputy if he would like to see the body and offered to show him.

As she opened the door for him, the deputy started across the threshold. Then he stepped back, visibly startled—and deeply moved. Here was a room ablaze with magnificent paintings and, in their midst, a beautiful oak casket with the deceased laid out with every possible offering of respect. Flowers surrounded him, candles burned, a Bible lay on the table where the last person had read for him. The man returned from the room shaken. Clearly, the one who had died was honored and revered. He called his superiors at the coroner's office, trying very hard to find the words to explain to them what he was witnessing and to find some way to put this bizarre situation into some official cubby hole that could make it work. There simply were none. The situation was off the chart. He was told they would have to remove the body.

But we were resolute. All through the tension-filled script being played out, our community group was absolutely united in our determination that Kim's wishes were going to be honored if there was any way we could possibly make it happen. The truth is, the whole thing was hilarious. We were in a play and taking turns at our moments on stage as if we had studied our parts for weeks. One character after another (and we were certainly an interesting group of characters) would step forward for his or her role in perfect coordination. Recalling the scene later, we all felt we were being exuberantly directed from the other side by two very involved and innovative playwrights, Kim and Ilse.

It was just the sort of drama Kim and Ilse loved. They had both thrived on stirring things up all their lives. Putting on "the performance" had always been foremost on their agenda! Ilse used to come into my college classes when I was teaching, and in minutes had commandeered bewildered students for a community play. She would sign them up for rehearsals before they knew what had happened. Furthermore, for years this pair of artists had criss-crossed the country in an old station wagon, stopping in towns to give workshops awash with color from Kim's paintings, which he created at the same time he mesmerized the audience with stories, while Ilse got everyone up and moving with eurythmy. Then together they would extol the joys of a spiritual path of knowledge.

Now the current drama went into the third act. Another actress stepped forth. She was a woman with dramatic capacities, and expansive gestures to accompany her words. Addressing the coroner's party with a breathless and fervent voice, she launched into an explanation of all the spiritual wonders that were taking place around this death. The two men on the couch were incredulous. But we had just bought about twenty minutes. Then one of the men turned to me and asked, "But why do you people do this?" So searching for a framework he could relate to, I tried to explain our philosophy. But frankly, in all fairness to him, it would be hard for anyone to make sense of why we were all gathered there creating beautiful funeral preparations in this home with none of Kim's relatives around to witness our efforts.

The gracious lady came through again and offered to order pizza for everyone. The coffin bearers rolled their eyes. It had been over two hours since they had arrived. Just as the final confrontation was shaping up, the dramatic actress, in a last ditch display, fell to her knees, hands clasped to her bosom, and pleaded with the men not to take away the body of our beloved Kim. The trio was speechless. The rest of us were pretty impressed too.

Just then the phone rang. It was Kim's sister, Emily, to the rescue. The conversation ensued that yes, she was his sister; yes, this is what he had ordered; yes, all was planned and paid for; and yes, she had the authority as a "blood relative" of the "official family" to say so.

Visibly relieved, the coroner's committee of three took their leave of us, the hefty men still shaking their heads. It just didn't make sense. Who was all the show for? The guy was dead and there was no one to impress. But I am quite confident none of them ever forgot this assignment. And I shall always remember the deep humanity of the deputy.

We did order pizza. We laughed. And we congratulated ourselves for our stunning performances to delay the removal. We had told the deputy we would stay the night to secure the home. Bill and I were the logical ones to do so. I teased Bill, that he was just an imposter as the executor because he hadn't been officially dubbed, so I said I was going to send an article to a national tabloid sheet saying that I had been forced to stay all night in a house with a "criminal and a dead body." It was community life in all its glory. Our dear, eighty-three-year-old Maulsby Kimball, went out with marvelous style.

Kim's sister, Emily, flew in for the funeral. She was overcome with gratitude for all we had done for her brother. When I closed the casket on the third day, I asked Emily to help. She was forever grateful to perform this last act of love for her beloved Kim, placing the silken cloth over his peaceful countenance and putting many flowers in the casket. Afterward, we stood together in prayerful silence.

Later, on Sunday, we had a last Advent celebration while Emily was still there. She was so glad we had brought the Christmas tree for Kim and put a golden angel on top. Baby Gabrielle toddled and chirped so sweetly between us as we sang and lit the candles on the tree. She looked at Emily with innocent brown eyes and smiled and then, somehow remembering the ceremony the week before, she went to the empty chair where Kim had been sitting last Sunday and put her favorite blanket there as an offering.

But the drama wasn't over yet. There was to be a brief ceremony with the priest at home before removing the body to the church for the funeral. I had called my daughter Mary to bring our green van for the transport and emphasized it had to be at nine in the morning. The timing was critical as not only did I have to get the casket and flowers arranged before the service, but I needed to set up several of Kim's paintings as well. But nine o'clock came and she was not there. Ten minutes passed.

Meanwhile at home, Mary was overcome with chagrin that the van was dusty and needed cleaning and furthermore, was nearly out of gas, hardly a proper hearse to honor a dear friend. She took the time to set things right. I had driven our old, brown pickup, with dinged fenders and an aging paint job down that morning. Mary still was not there. Okay, we would take the truck. The surprised friends who carried out the body did what I asked and put the casket in the pickup bed. I flung a blanket over it and we hastily roped it down. I climbed in the driver's seat and, wheels spinning in the gravel, headed out only to nearly collide head on with Mary who was coming in the driveway. "We can transfer it," she shouted to me, but I shook my head and roared on down the street. Every minute counted now. My artistic senses fully aflame, I knew it just wouldn't do to be running around setting things up while people were coming in for the service. I had a young man with me. To this day he looks at me with awe about that trip, whizzing over bumps, bridges and highways to the church in what was surely "Mr. Toad's Wild Ride" taken to new level! Or, as the old song says "Get me to the church on time." I think Kim liked that part too.

The sanctuary was filled, with standing room only. It was December 21st, the winter solstice. This benevolent man was deeply loved by young and old alike. Everyone felt it a real honor to say they were a friend of Kim's.

During the service, the deeper meaning of Kim's last words dawned for me. Kim had a very developed wit and sense of humor, including a rare ability to play on words. Now I sensed the double meaning in his last message. When he saw the rose, he had cried out, "That is very fine indeed!" One can look at a rose in many ways; as a symbol of eternal beauty, of sacrifice, or of universal love and peace. In this case, I believe Kim's words about the rose are his challenge to anyone on a spiritual path, that is to take all these things that the rose can mean in life, and put them into deeds. In other words, "That is very fine—**in deed**!"

I am humbled and honored to have the rare gift Kim gave me with his death. His loving influence lives on in countless lives he touched, not just my own. But it was my privilege to experience the union, the spiritual teamwork, the lifting and leaving of the spirit from an old body into the light, and the sense of mystical angelic accompaniment. That shall always be with me.

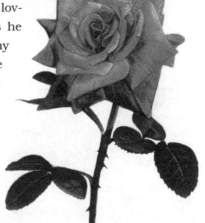

"The rose is very fine—in deed."

213

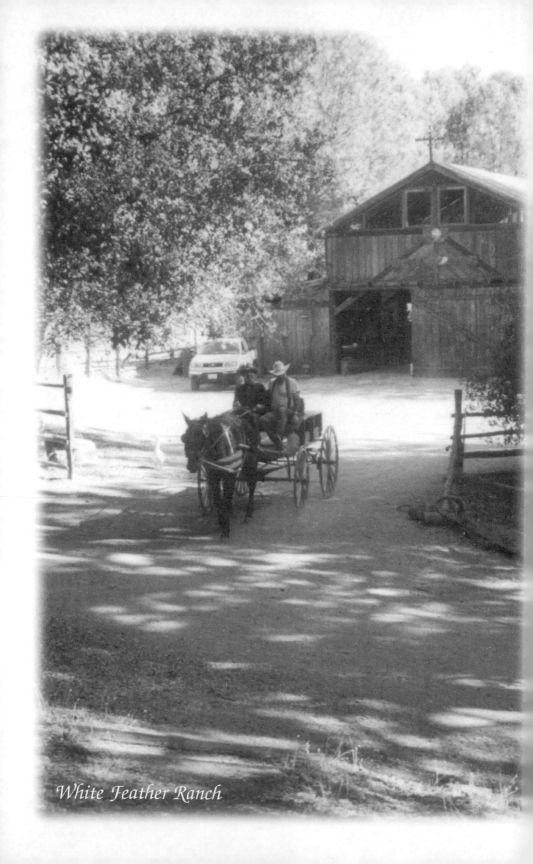

White Feather Ranch

FUTURE COMMUNITY

We gathered at our home, White Feather Ranch, at Easter time. It was a group of individuals seemingly brought together at random. Two of our children and their families were there, but all the others were unrelated friends. Yet we soon realized that everyone present had recently experienced the loss of loved ones. We were a multi-ethnic group, eclectic in religious views and spanning four generations, from a babe and young children to grandparents. In seven days, this constellation of souls, in the most natural way, created a vibrant and tangible interweaving with souls living on the other side of the threshold. At the end of that time, I became aware of what had happened and what such sharing can mean as an archetype for community of the future.

Our lovely daughter-in-law, Carolyn, Cameron's wife, was there. When she was four months pregnant with her first child, her father died. She and Cameron flew back to her family home before his passing, and, at her father's bidding, made the casket for him. His death was expected. But her mother's was not. Two weeks before her baby was born, her mother suddenly died. It was unbelievable sorrow to bear.

There was Rose, who was just thirteen, and her father. His wife, Rose's wonderful, dynamic mother who had been a very close friend to most of us, had died so rapidly with cancer it left everyone stunned. My husband's brother had crossed with cancer that year, almost as quickly.

Joaquin was eleven. His father was a native Californian of Mexican heritage. He had died when his son was a babe. Joaquin was visiting as a companion for my grandson, Alex. Joaquin's best friend, eight-year-old Jake, had recently died after a fall from a tree where he was playing.

Chie was from Japan, and had no close blood family. When her baby boy, Yasuhiro, was only two weeks old, her mother was murdered. On the day the criminal was brought to trial, she found her baby had Tay Sach's, a fatal disease. With unwavering love, she had nurtured Yasuhiro, to live two years beyond the normally expected life span for a child with such an illness. In that time, she learned quiet soul ways to communicate with her child, who was totally helpless and could not speak.

Terry was there with her sunshine delight of a young toddler, Timothy. His older sister, Emily, had died of leukemia when he was four months old. This was the first time Terry met Chie. Timothy would inherit Yasuhiro's teddy bear hat. Another friend, Mary, and her two young children also joined us. She was preparing; a difficult death, where her spiritual awareness would make all the difference, would occur a little over a year later.

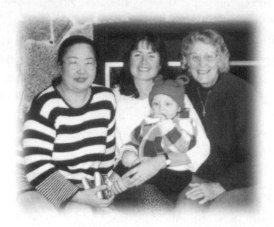

At first description, it sounds like the gathering of a mournful crew. It was anything but that. These were people who had gone to the core of life through sorrow and loss and had come back with the courage to pronounce that life, while incredibly hard, is good. There were no façades, everyone was authentic. Everyone was present, real. Life was too precious to be anything else. That awareness wove through the group as common, unspoken knowledge.

Of course, we ate a lot. Meals were abundant and snacks ongoing. Food grown on the ranch was a hearty basis for the fare. Everyone did his or her part. We talked, we slept, we walked, we read, and we played. We had a baseball game in the front pasture in honor of Jake, who had loved the sport. There were vigorous and playful challenges at the basketball hoop in the barn. We had rousing, competitive pool games, and bouts of Pictionary played with rowdy, shrieking whoops of laughter. There was virtually no television. All seven of the children had come from homes where media did not rule, and just enjoying each other was the important thing.

We took walks to the granite rocks to watch the sunsets together and reveled in sparkling stars at night. Mary's little four-year-old daughter lavished daily affection on the baby geese. We took rides on the ancient flatbed truck, the uncomplicated chugs and putts of the seventy-year-old engine making a comforting sound as we rolled over the hills. We sat in big circles and gave each other shoulder rubs and foot rubs. We sang, we prayed, and laughed. There was a whole lot of laughing and joking. Clusters of twos and threes formed for visiting and sharing, then dissolved and reformed in an easy exchange of intergenerational interests and all blessed with the poignancy and joy of life. The healthy soul must weep and laugh, in-breathing and out-breathing. We were together for healing and health.

Anyone could shed tears at any time and it was okay. Anyone could talk freely about his or her special loved one at any time—and everyone listened. Joaquin, standing tall, straight and serious, recited Jake's birthday verse which his teacher had prophetically given Jake when he was seven, the year before he died. Joaquin had memorized it.

JACOB'S SECOND GRADE BIRTHDAY VERSE

I have lived with the winds, with the clouds and the showers

I have harkened to speech without words

I have joyed to the joy of the blossoming flowers

And joined the sweet song of the birds.

I have danced to the dance that all nature is dancing

The hedgehog so serious, the wild pony prancing

Ah, life, lovely life, you are young and entrancing

But the stars gleaming down on me waken me now

To their strong, silent speech I must listen somehow.

We all felt so proud of this young boy and the beautiful, unabashed love with which he offered the poem. It brought tears to all our eyes. He would later go on to recite it with perfect poise in many, many places, his on-going tribute to his beloved friend.

The teenaged grand daughters planned our Easter sunrise service. They made elaborate programs and picked the hymns to be sung. Prayers and Bible readings were planned and put in the program books.

In the dark before Easter dawn, there was a round of knocking on bedroom doors, the gentle shaking of shoulders of children sleeping dorm-style across the floors and whispered greetings to awaken everyone. We all gradually assembled, sleepy-eyed but eager. It is our tradition to walk in silence the quarter-mile down to the spring that flows from under the old cedar tree in the forest. The only sounds as the group walked to the woods through the mists of morning were the crunch of our shoes on the gravel road and the birds awakening to the coming dawn. At the spring, we took a few drops of Easter new water and sang together. Then we climbed up to the hill through the soft white mists to stand before the rising sun as it shone through the swirling veils of clouds.

The service was deep and emotional. We all could speak of our loved one in any way we were moved to share. The culminating moment came when Rose and Gabrielle read the passages from the Bible describing Christ's resurrection . . . "and the stone was rolled away . . . He is risen" It was all there—the sorrow, the loss, the hope, the resurrection. Most of that week, we were thirteen in number, but we were multitudes. We all had no doubt of that. What made this gathering new and different, and the reason I feel it was an archetype for meetings of such groups in the future, was the mutual awareness of the vital spiritual presence of those who had died. Virtually every conversation was sprinkled with reference to one of them, with good memories of them. Those living in spirit fit in as easily, as naturally, and as continuously, as if they were making their contributions in person among us.

I believe the day will come when people, working together, will realize and acknowledge in an everyday, matter-of-fact way, that loved ones in the spirit are always present in our lives and caring about us. They are bringing us together. They are loving us from the other side. They are hoping we will find our mission to help the world, and they hope for, and need, our prayers and spiritual thoughts for their well-being and their journeys. I believe if we could truly see the power, the extent, the expansive reach of the web of creative community life between heaven and earth, we would all be truly amazed. Such tremendous spiritual love and inspiration and guidance from angelic realms and from our loved ones on the other side pours into our lives when we can receive it. It is an endless source of inspiration, strength, and hope to give us words to say, gestures to make and deeds to do. Truly will "the circle be unbroken" as we realize that in caring for one another, we are carried by the spiritual world, the angels, and those we loved in this life and the next . . . the new community of the future.

In The Light of A Child, Michael Hedley Burton

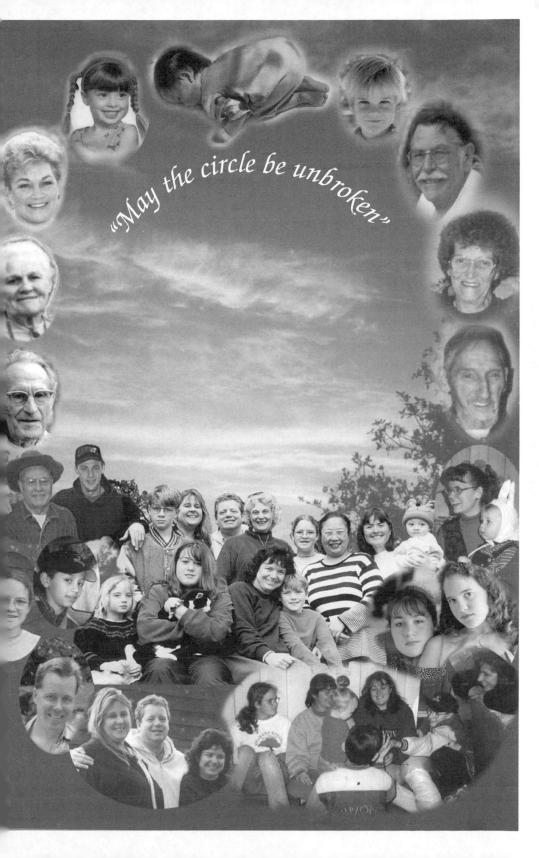

"May the circle be unbroken"

BIBLIOGRAPHY

Atwater, P.M.H., *Coming Back to Life, The After Effects of the Near Death Experience*, Toronto, Ballantine books, 1992

Barnes, Christy, & Janet Hutchinson, *The Uprising in Dying, Words and Verses For Those Close to the Experience Surrounding The Threshold of Death*, New York, Adonis Press, 1990 **(A beautiful collection of verses for the dying and for supporting spiritual connections to those who have died)**

Bernard, Jan, R.N. N.D. and Schneider, Miriam, RN CRNH, *The True Work of Dying, A Practical and Compassionate Guide to Easing the Death Process*, New York, Avon Books,1996

Brinkley, Dannion, *Saved By the Light*, New York, Villard Press, 1994 **(A man with two near death experiences)**

Brinkley, Dannion, with Paul Perry, *At Peace in the Light*, New York, Harper Collins Pub. 1995

Callanan, Maggie, and Kelley, Patricia, *Final Gifts, Understanding the Special Awareness, Needs and Communications of the Dying*, New York, Poseidon Press, 1992 **(An excellent book for enhancing understanding of the dying individual)**

Callari, Elizabeth, *A Gentle Death, Personal Caregiving to the Terminally Ill*

Capel, Evelyn Francis, *Death, The End is the Beginning*, London, Christian Community Press, 1979

Carlson Lisa, *Caring For The Dead, Your Final Act of Love, A Complete Guide for those Making Funeral Arrangements With or Without a Funeral Director*, Vermont, Upper Access Publishers, 1998 **(This book gives legal requirements for home death in all states and is the most comprehensive guide for current funeral issues.)**

Chaney, Earlyne, *The Mystery of Death and Dying*, York Beach, Maine, Samuel Weiser, Inc. 1988

Childs, Dr. Gilbert and Sylvia, *The Journey Continues, Finding A New Relationship to Death*, London, Sophia Books, Rudolf Steiner Press, 1998

Cornish, John, *About Death and After*, Sussex, England, New Knowledge Books, 1975

Dass, Ram, Paul Gorman, *How Can I Help? Stories and Reflections on Service*, New York, Alfred A. Knopf, 1991

Dass, Ram, *Still Here*, New York, Riverhead Books, 2001

Davies, Phyllis, *Grief, Climb Toward Understanding,* San Luis Obispo. CA, Sunnybank Publishers, 1988

DePaola, Tome *Nana Upstairs, Nana Downstairs,* New York, Viking Penguin Books, 1973 **(for children)**

Deverell, Dore, *Light Beyond The Darkness,* London, Temple Lodge Press, 1996 **(A mother's story of reading to her son after his suicide and their spiritual connection)**

Doore, Gary, Ph.D.,Editor, *What Survives? Contemporary Explorations of Life After Death,* New York, St. Martin's Press, 1990

Drake, Stanley, *Though You Die,* Floris Books, Edinburgh, 1988 **(Clear insightful spiritual view)**

Duda, Deborah, *Coming Home, A Guide to Dying at Home With Dignity,* New York, Aurora Press, 1987 **(Comprehensive practical guide for home death care with a spiritual perspective)**

Eadie, Betty J., *Embraced By The Light,* Placerville, CA, Gold Leaf Press, 1992

Farr, Sidney Saylor, *What Tom Sawyer Learned from Dying,* Norfolk, VA, Hampton Roads Publishing, 1993

Fremantle Francesca and Chogyam Trungpa, *The Tibetan Book of The Dead, The Great Liberation Through Hearing in the Bardo,* Boston, London, 1987 Shambala

Gill, Derek, *Quest, The Life of Elizabeth Kubler-Ross,* Toronto, Harper and Row, 1980

Glas, Norbert, M.D., *The Fulfillment of Old Age,* New York, Anthroposophic Press, Inc., 1970 **(An excellent book on the challenges of aging and a spiritual view of preparation for death)**

Greaves, Helen, *Testimony of Light,* Great Britain, Hillman Printers Ltd.,1969

Grollman, Earl, *Living When A Loved One Has Died,* Boston, Beacon Press, 1977

Guggenheim, Bill and Judy, *Hello From Heaven,* New York, Bantam Books, 1995

Hains, Barbara, and Bascom, Lionel, *Full Circle, The Near Death Experience and Beyond,* New York, Pocket Books, Simon and Schuster, 1990

Heavilin, Marilyn, *Roses In December, Finding Strength in Grief,* San Bernadino, CA, Here's Life Publishers, 1986

Heisler, Rev. Hermann, *Our Relationship to Those Who Have Died,* New York, St. George Press, 1976

Hodson, Geoffrey, *Through The Gateway of Death,* Wheaton, Illinois, Theosophical Publishing House, 1953

Hogan, Pat, *Alison's Gift,* New York, Touchstone Books, 1997 **(A beautiful book of honoring a child's death with a home vigil)**

Humann, Harvey, *Death Without Fear,* Lawrence, Kansas, Penthe Publishing Co., 1992

Hunter, Rev. John, *Help In Dying,* New York, Christian Community, 1967

Jocelyn, Beredene, *Citizens of the Cosmos, Life's Unfolding from Conception through Death to Rebirth,* New York, Continuum Pub., 1981 **(in-depth spiritual view of life cycles)**

Jury, Mark and Dan, *Gramp,* New York, Viking Press, 1976

Krementz, Jill, *How It Feels When a Parent Dies,* New York, Alfred A. Knopf, 1991

(Below are books by Elisabeth Kubler-Ross, pioneer in death and dying in America—her books are classics on the subject.)

Kubler-Ross, Elisabeth, *Death, The Final Stage of Growth,* New Jersey, Prenctice Hall, 1975

Kubler-Ross, Elisabeth, *Living With Death And Dying,* New York, McMillan Publishing, 1981

Kubler-Ross, Elisabeth, *On Death and Dying,* New York, McMillan Publishing, 1969

Kubler-Ross, Elisabeth, *On Children and Death,* New York, McMillan Publishing, 1983

Kubler-Ross, Elisabeth, *Questions and Answers on Death and Dying,* New York, McMillan Publishing, 1974

Kubler-Ross, Elisabeth, *Remember the Secret,* Berkeley, Celestial Arts, 1982 **(for children)**

Kubler-Ross, Elisabeth, *To Live Until We Say Goodbye,* New Jersey, Prentice Hall Publishing, 1978

Kubler-Ross, Elisabeth, *Working It Through,* New York, McMillan Publishing, 1982

Kubler-Ross, Elisabeth, *Aids, The Ultimate Challenge*, New York, McMillan Publishing, 1987

Kubler-Ross, Elisabeth, *On Life After Death*, Berkeley, Celestial Arts, 1991

Kubler-Ross, Elisabeth *The Wheel of Life, A Memoir of Living and Dying*, New York, Scribner, 1997

Kubler-Ross, Elizabeth and David Kessler, *Life Lessons*, New York, Scribner, 2000

Kushner, Harold, *When Bad Things Happen to Good People*, New York, Avon Books, 1981

Kyber, Manfred, *Three Candles of Little Veronica, A Classic Story of a Child's Soul in This World and the Next*, Berkeley, CA.,Celestial Arts, **(a classic for adults and children)**

LaConte, Ellen, *On Light Alone, A Guru Meditation on the Good Death of Helen Nearing*, Stockton Springs, Maine, Loose Leaf Press, 1996

(The following are books by Stephen Levine, nationally known counselor in death and dying)

Levine, Stephen, *A Gradual Awakening*, New York, Anchor Press/Doubleday, 1984

Levine, Stephen, *Healing Into Life and Death*, New York, Anchor Press, Doubleday, 1987

Levine, Stephen, *Meetings At The Edge, Dialogues With the Grieving and the Dying, the Healing and the Healed*, New York, Anchor Press, Doubleday, 1984

Levine, Stephen, *Who Dies?, An Investigation of Conscious Living and Conscious Dying*, New York, Anchor Press, Doubleday, 1982

Levine, Stephen, *Guided Meditations, Explorations and Healings*, New York, Anchor Press, Doubleday, 1991

Levine, Stephen, *How To Live This Year As If It Were Your Last*, New York, McMillan Library, 1998

Lewis, C. S., *A Grief Observed*, New York, Bantam Books, 1976 **(A very insightful book on experiencing a loved one across the threshold)**

Lewis, Rev. Richard (and others), *Help For Those Whose Children Have Died*, 3548 Eisenhower Drive, Sacramento, CA. 95826, 1998

Lievegoed, Bernard, *Man On The Threshold*, **(includes in-depth spiritual explanation of the double.)**

Lonsdale, Elias, Theanna, *The Book of Theanna, In the Lands that Follow Death,* Berkeley, CA., Frog, Ltd. 1993

Lyons, Jerri and Va Melvin, Janelle, **Handbook For Creating A Home Funeral,** Sebastopol, CA 1998, www.finalpassages.org.

Mayer, Gladys, *Behind The Veils of Death and Sleep,* Sussex, England, New Knowledge Books

Mitford, Jessica, *The American Way of Death,* New York, Simon and Shuster, 1963

Moody, Raymond, M.D., *Life After Life,* New York, Bantam Books, Inc. 1975 **(The first major book on case studies of near death experiences)**

Moody, Raymond, M.D. *Reflections on Life After Life,* New York, Bantam Books, Inc. 1977

Moody, Raymond, M.D. *The Light Beyond,* New York, Bantam Books, Inc. 1989

Morse, Melvin, M.D. *Closer To the Light, Learning From the Near Death Experiences of Children,* New York, Ivy Books, Ballantine, 1990

Morse, Melvin, M.D. and Paul Perry, *Transformed by the Light, the Powerful Effect of Near Death Experiences on People's Lives,* New York, Villiard Books, Random House, Inc., 1992

Murphet, Howard, *Beyond Death, The Undiscovered Country,* Wheaton, Illinois, Theosophical Publishing House, 1984

Panuthos, Claudia and Romeo, Catherine, *Ended Beginnings, Healing Childbearing Losses,* New York, Warner Books, 1984

Parrish-Harra, Carol W. *A New Age Handbook on Death and Dying,* Marina del Rey, CA. DeVorss & Co., 1982 **(A very well done practical spiritual guide)**

Poppelbaum, Harmann, *Man's Eternal Biography,* Spring Valley, New York, Adonis Press, 1943

Priever, Werner, M.D. *Illness and the Double,* Spring Valley, New York, Mercury Press, 1982

Puryear Ann, *Steven Lives, His Life of Suicide and After Life,* Scottsdale, Arizona, 1993 New Paradigm Press

Rinpoche, Sogyal, *The Tibetan Book of Living and Dying,* San Francisco, Harper, 1994

Ring, Kenneth, M.D., *Healing Toward Omega, In Search of the Meaning of Near Death Experience*, New York, Morrow Publishing, 1985

Ring, Kenneth, M.D. *Life At Death, A Scientific Investigation of the Near Death Experience*, New York, Morrow Publishing, 1982

Ritchie, George G., M.D. (with Elizabeth Sherrill), *Return from Tomorrow*, New York, Chosen Books, Revell Co., 1978 **(The first major extensive near death experience of an imminent psychiatrist from WW II—published in America.)**

Ritchie, George G. M.D., *My Life After Dying, Becoming Alive to Universal Love*, Norwalk, VA., Hampton Roads Publishing, 1991

Roseberry, Salli, Watanabi, Carol, *The Art of Dying, Honoring and Celebrating Life's Passages*, Berkeley, CA., Celestial Arts, 2001

Rosof, Barbara, *The Worst Loss, How Families Heal From the Death of a Child*, New York, Henry Holt & Co., 1994

Rozell, Calvert, *The Near Death Experience, In the Light of Scientific The Research and the Spiritual Science of Rudolf Steiner*, New York, Anthroposophic Press, 1992 **(An excellent combination of scientific and metaphysical research into near death experience.)**

Sabom, Michael, M.D., *Recollections of Death, A Medical Investigation*, New York, Harper and Row, 1982

Sankar, Andrea, *Dying At Home, A Family Guide for Caregiving*, Baltimore, John Hopkins University Press, 1991, **(A comprehensive guide for caring for the dying at home)**

Schilling, Karin V., *Where Are You? The Death of My Child*, New York, Anthroposophic Press 1988 **(Excellent book on living through the loss of a child with the overview of spiritual knowledge)**

Schoeneck, Therese, *Hope for the Bereaved, Understanding, Coping and Growing Through Grief*, New York, Hope for the Bereaved, 1995 (Excellent handbook of articles and poems written by bereaved people)

(The following books give a deep spiritual scientific view of the human experience beyond death)

Steiner, Rudolf, *Staying Connected, How To Continue Your Relationship to Those Who Have Died*, Hudson, New York, Anthroposophic Press, 1999

Steiner, Rudolf, *The Dead Are With Us*, London, Rudolf Steiner Press, 1985

Steiner, Rudolf, *Links Between the Living and the Dead*, London, Anthroposophic Press, 1960 (out of print)

Steiner, Rudolf, *Theosophy, An Introduction to the Supersensible Knowledge of the World and Destination of Man,* New York, Anthroposophic Press, 1971

Steiner, Rudolf, *Life Between Death and Rebirth,* New York, Anthroposophic Press, 1985

Steiner, Rudolf, *Earthly Death and Cosmic Life,* New York, Garber Communications, Anthroposophic Press, 1989

Steiner, Rudolf, *The Forming of Destiny and Life After Death,* Garber Communications, Anthroposophic Press, 1989

Steiner, Rudolf, *The Presence of the Dead on the Spiritual Path,* New York, Anthroposophic Press, 1990

Steiner, Rudolf, *Geographic Medicine,* Spring Valley, New York, Mercury Press, 1979

Stoddar, Sandol, *The Hospice Movement, A Better Way of Caring for the Dying,* New York, Vintage Books, Random House, 1978

Sturgeon-Day, Lee, *A Slice of Life, A Personal Story of Healing Through Cancer,* Royal Oak, MI, Lifeways, 1991

Sturgeon-Day, Lee, *Double Trouble WorkBook,* P. O. Box 2922 Prescott, AZ. 8630l, Lifeways, Bitesize Books, 1999 **(Insights into the double)**

Tatelbaum, Judy, *The Courage to Grieve, Creative Living, Recovery and Growth Through Grief,* New York, Harper and Row, 1980

Wetzl, Joseph, (editor-translator) *The Bridge Over the River, Communications from Life After Death of a Young Artist Who Died in WW1,* New York, Anthroposophic Press, 1974

The Thanks-Be-To-Grandmother-Winifred Foundation contributed support for this bibliography.

ABOUT THE AUTHOR

Nancy Jewel Poer was born and raised in California. As a child she loved horses and outdoor life and graduated from the University of Arizona with hopes of becoming a veterinarian. But her large family of six children, three sons and three daughters, became the creative center of her work, along with teaching in the International Waldorf schools.

Nancy is known across the United States, for her lively lectures on Waldorf education, parenting, child development, the spiritual feminine and the role of women in America, and threshold work. She felt called to threshold work, first assisting with births, and then pioneering support with home deaths in the community, which she has done for the past twenty-five years. She has helped in the founding of threshold groups throughout the country. An artist as well as a writer, she has published *A Child's First Book* and art prints for children.

She is co-founder of Rudolft Steiner College, a Waldorf teachers' college near Sacramento, and has taught there for twenty-eight years. Prior to that she taught children at all grade levels, K-12, and began three kindergartens, the last as the founding teacher for the Cedar Springs Waldorf School in Placerville, California.

She lives with her husband of many decades in the Sierra foothills on White Feather ranch where they raise cattle, have a bio-dynamic garden, sponsor youth conferences, and Nancy gives women's retreats and threshold conferences to help pass the work on to others.

*"The name of death was never
terrible to him that knew to live."*

Ralph Waldo Emerson